Ceremonial Chemistry

THE RITUAL PERSECUTION OF DRUGS, ADDICTS, AND PUSHERS

Thomas Szasz

Revised Edition

LP Learning Publications, Inc.
Holmes Beach, Florida

Library of Congress Cataloging in Publication Data

Szasz, Thomas Stephen, 1920-
    Ceremonial chemistry.

    Bibliography: p.
    Includes index.
    1. drug abuse — United States.   2. Social control.
3. Narcotics, Control of — United States.
I. Title
HV5825.S95   1985   363.4'5'0973   84-40733
ISBN 1-55691-019-3 (lib./bdg.)

Learning Publications, Inc.
5351 Gulf Drive
P.O. Box 1338
Holmes Beach, FL 34218-1338

Cover Design by Barbara Wirtz

Printing: 8 7 6 5   Year: 9 8 7 6

Printed and bound in the United States of America.

Men are qualified for civil liberty in exact proportion to their disposition to put moral chains upon their own appetites; in proportion as their love of justice is above their rapacity; in proportion as their soundness and sobriety of understanding is above their vanity and presumption; in proportion as they are more disposed to listen to the counsels of the wise and good, in preference to the flattery of knaves. Society cannot exist unless a controlling power upon will and appetite be placed somewhere, and the less of it there is within, the more there must be without. It is ordained in the eternal constitution of things, that men of intemperate minds cannot be free. Their passions forge their fetters.

EDMUND BURKE (1791)

Contributing Editor
Edsel L. Erickson

ACKNOWLEDGMENTS

With each new book, my debt and gratitude to my brother George expand. His devotion to my work is beyond praise, and any effort to acknowledge it is bound to be inadequate. I wish to thank also my daughters, Margot and Susan Marie, for their generous efforts in locating source materials, their tough-minded scrutiny of my views, and their fresh ideas; Bill Whitehead, my editor at Doubleday, for his continuing conscientious assistance with my books, and in particular with this one; my colleague Ronald Carino, for reading the entire manuscript and for many suggestions for revision; Helen Vermeychuk, for advice and guidance with respect to Greek sources and terminology; the staff of the Library of the State University of New York, Upstate Medical Center, for untiring efforts to secure many of the references consulted in the preparation of this volume; and my secretary, Debbie Murphy, for her careful and efficient labors.

CONTENTS

PREFACE

There is probably one thing, and one thing only, on which the leaders of all modern states agree; on which Catholics, Protestants, Jews, Mohammedans, and atheists agree; on which Democrats, Republicans, Socialists, Communists, Liberals, and Conservatives agree; on which medical and scientific authorities throughout the world agree; and on which the views, as expressed through opinion polls and voting records, of the large majority of individuals in all civilized countries agree. That thing is the "scientific fact" that certain substances which people like to ingest or inject are "dangerous" both to those who use them and to others; and that the use of such substances constitutes "drug abuse" or "drug addiction"—a disease whose control and eradication are the duty of the combined forces of the medical profession and the state. However, there is little agreement—from people to people, country to country, even decade to decade—on which substances are acceptable and their use therefore considered a popular pastime, and which substances are unacceptable and their use therefore considered "drug abuse" and "drug addiction."

My aim in this book is at once simple and sweeping. First, I wish to identify the actual occurrences that constitute our so-called drug problem. I shall show that these phenomena in fact consist of the passionate promotion and panicky prohibition of various substances; the habitual use and the dreaded avoidance of certain drugs; and, most generally, the regulation—by language, law, custom, religion, and every other conceivable means of social and symbolic control—of certain kinds of ceremonial and sumptuary behaviors.

Second, I wish to identify the conceptual realm and logical class into which these phenomena belong. I shall show that they belong in the realm of religion and politics; that "dangerous drugs," addicts, and pushers are the scapegoats of our modern, secular, therapeutically imbued societies; and that the ritual persecution of these pharmacological and human agents must be seen against the historical backdrop of the ritual persecution of other scapegoats, such as witches, Jews, and madmen.

And third, I wish to identify the moral and legal implications of the view that using and avoiding drugs are not matters of health and disease but matters of good and evil; that, in other words, drug abuse is not a regrettable medical disease but a repudiated religious observance. Accordingly, our options with respect to the "problem" of drugs are the same as our options with respect to the "problem" of religions: that is, we can practice various degrees of tolerance and intolerance toward those whose religions —whether theocratic or therapeutic—differ from our own.

For the past half-century the American people have engaged in one of the most ruthless wars—fought under the colors of drugs and doctors, diseases and treatments—that the world has ever seen. If a hundred years ago the American government had tried to regulate what substances its citizens could or could not ingest, the effort would have been ridiculed as absurd and rejected as unconstitutional. If fifty years ago the American government had tried to regulate what crops farmers in foreign countries could or could not cultivate, the effort would have been criticized as meddling and rejected as colonialism. Yet now the American government is deeply committed to imposing precisely such regulations—on its own citizens by means of criminal and mental health laws, and on those of other countries by means of economic threats and incentives; and these regulations—called "drug controls" or "narcotic controls"—are hailed and supported by countless individuals and institutions, both at home and abroad.

We have thus managed to replace racial, religious, and military coercions and colonialisms, which now seem to us dishonorable, with medical and therapeutic coercions and colonialisms, which now seem to us honorable. Because these latter controls are ostensibly based on Science and aim to secure only Health, and because those who are so coerced and colonized often worship the idols of medical and therapeutic scientism as ardently as do the coercers and colonizers, the victims cannot even articulate their predicament and are therefore quite powerless to resist their victimizers. Perhaps such preying of people upon people—such symbolic cannibalism, providing meaning for one life by depriving another of meaning—is an inexorable part of the human condition and is therefore inevitable. But it is surely not inevitable for any one person to deceive himself or herself into believing that the ritual persecutions of scapegoats—in Crusades, Inquisitions, Final Solutions, or Wars on Drug Abuse—actually propitiate deities or prevent diseases.

THOMAS SZASZ

Syracuse, New York
September 1, 1973

PREFACE TO THE 1985 EDITION

More than a decade has passed since I wrote the Preface to the original edition of this book. Many things in American life have changed during these years, but the "war on drugs" is not one of them. With respect to "drug abuse" and "drug policies," everything is the same, only, to put it colloquially, more so. Countless Americans continue to grow and smuggle, sell and buy, ingest, inhale, and inject illicit drugs in seemingly ever-increasing quantities. Others—or perhaps some of the same ones—continue to agitate against "drug abuse" and the "drug traffic" with seemingly ever-increasing imbecility and intensity. All the while the ordinary American is increasingly endangered in his daily life, both by those who "abuse" drugs and by those whose job it is to abuse "drug abusers."

Yet, none of this makes people doubt the validity of their premises concerning our so-called "drug problem" or the legitimacy of the social policies ostensibly aimed at combating it. Indeed, why should it? If people want to deny that the danger in "dangerous drugs"—such as heroin, cocaine, or marijuana—lies not in the substances themselves but in the human propensity to take them and in the personal decisions of those who use them, then they will deny it. And, having denied it, they will proceed to lose sight of such old-fashioned but eternally valid ideas as temptation and self-control, and will end up denying the reality of personal freedom and responsibility as well. Finally, people will convince themselves—as most Americans have—that our "drug problem" is something historically novel, involving new diseases requiring new treatments. This is a costly illusion.

Supposedly, the great moral contest of our age is the struggle between communism and capitalism. Actually, that struggle conceals an even greater contest—a struggle waged by politicians and their intellectual lackeys, both East and West, against free will and personal responsibility. Whether couched in the imagery of historical or biological determinism, whether seen as Marxist or behavioral "science," the real message is the same: the individual is not responsible for his behavior; he is a victim who must be saved (from capitalism or "drugs") by a protective, therapeutic state.

The simple fact is that, so long as they remain in the laboratory or on the shelf—that is, anywhere outside of the human body—drugs are merely inert substances. Heroin, cocaine, and marijuana pose no problems for those who do not take them, and, unlike the currently fashionable "psychiatric drugs," no one is forced to take them. Hence, it is a grave abuse of language to call certain (illicit) drugs "dangerous," and it is worse than folly to declare "war" on them.

Thomas Szasz

Syracuse, New York
November 1, 1984

INTRODUCTION

In its present popular and professional use, the term "addiction" refers not to a disease but to a despised kind of deviance. Hence the term "addict" refers not to a bona fide patient but to a stigmatized identity, usually stamped on a person against his or her will. Addiction (or drug abuse) thus resembles mental illness and witchcraft, and the addict (or drug abuser) resembles the mental patient and witch, inasmuch as all of these names identify categories of deviance and their occupants. Indeed, it would be more precise to say that addiction is considered to be a specific mental illness, just as hysteria, depression, and schizophrenia are considered to be other specific mental illnesses.

Accordingly, the observations and arguments about mental illness and the psychiatric enterprise which I have offered elsewhere—especially in *The Myth of Mental Illness* and *The Manufacture of Madness*—apply, *mutatis mutandis,* to addiction, addicts, and the so-called experts who profess to labor ceaselessly and selflessly on their behalf.[1] I will try not to repeat these observations and arguments here, and to confine myself, so far as possible, to those aspects of drug use and the persecutions of drug users that characterize these behaviors and distinguish them from other types of medically defined deviance and their psychiatric persecutions.

The ideal witch was initially a weird woman, the ideal madman a murderous maniac, and the ideal addict a deranged dope fiend; but once these categories became accepted as not only real but immensely important, the ranks from which such deviants could be recruited grew rapidly. Eventually anyone—save perhaps the most successful deviant mongers and their most powerful masters—could be "discovered" to be a witch, a madman, or a drug abuser; and witchcraft, insanity, and drug abuse were then declared to be "plagues" of "epidemic proportions" from whose "infection" no one was immune.

In the case of addiction mongering, three intertwining mechanisms for creating and discovering "addiction-prone" persons may be distinguished. The first is the classification, as "dangerous narcotics," of certain substances which are neither dangerous nor narcotic, but which are particularly popular with groups whose members readily lend themselves to social and psychiatric stigmatization (such substances being marijuana and amphetamines, and such groups being the metropolitan blacks and Puerto Ricans, and the young). The second is the prohibition of these substances and the persecution—through corrupt and capricious law enforcement—of those associated with their use, as bad criminals ("pushers") and as mad patients ("addicts" and "dope fiends"). The third mechanism is the persistent claim that the use of "dangerous narcotics" is increasing at an alarming rate, thus waging, in effect, a gigantic advertising campaign for the use of drugs that, although illegal, are readily available through illicit channels and are supposedly the source of immense "pleasures." These processes insure a limitless source of "raw materials" out of which officially accredited and labeled addicts may be manufactured as needed.

As the Christian West once confronted the problem of witchcraft, so now the Scientific World confronts the problem of drugcraft. The one had been as much the product of its own creation as is now the other. The manufacture of the "drug problem" does, however, generate certain phenomena which could be described or dealt with in a number of ways. Many of these phenomena—especially the prohibition of certain substances called "dangerous drugs" and their use called "drug abuse" or "drug addiction"—are now discussed in textbooks of pharmacology. This is as if the use of holy water were discussed in textbooks of inorganic chemistry. For if the study of drug addiction belongs to pharmacology because addiction has to do with drugs, then the study of baptism belongs to inorganic chemistry because this ceremony has to do with water.

Baptism is, of course, a ceremony and is generally recognized as such. Many kinds of drug use—for example, certain types of self-medication—also constitute ceremonies, but are not so recognized. Accordingly, the study of ceremonial drug use belongs to anthropology and religion, rather than to pharmacology and medicine, and should properly be called "ceremonial chemistry." I propose, in other words, that we distinguish more sharply than we have heretofore between the study of drugs and the study of drug use and drug avoidance. Organic chemistry, biological chemistry, and pharmacology are all concerned with the chemical properties and biological effects of *drugs*. Ceremonial chemistry, on the other hand, is concerned with the personal and cultural circumstances of *drug use* and *drug avoidance*. The subject matter of ceremonial chemistry is thus the magical as opposed to the medical, the ritual as opposed to the technical dimensions of drug use; more specifically, it is the approval and disapproval, promotion and prohibition, use and avoidance of symbolically significant substances, and the explanations and justifications offered for the consequences and control of their employment.

Addictive drugs stand in the same sort of relation to ordinary or non-addictive drugs as holy water stands in relation to ordinary or non-holy water. Once we identify certain drugs, call them "addictive," and place them in the same class with other drugs, such as antibiotics, diuretics, hormones, and so forth, we commit a category error similar to that which we would commit if we distinguished a type of water called "holy" and placed it in the same class with distilled water or heavy water.[2] It follows, then, that trying to understand drug addiction by studying drugs makes about as much sense as trying to understand holy water by studying water; and that regulating the use of addictive drugs by the kinds of drugs they are, makes as much sense as regulating the use of holy water by the kind of water it is.

Yet this is just what we do now. The confusion we thus generate—in our own minds and lives, and in the minds and lives of those we touch through our legislation, treatment, or "common sense"—could not be greater. For the folly into which we have fallen is of truly gigantic proportion: we have dethroned God and the devil, and have replaced them with new gods and devils. Our new gods and devils—our own creations, but mysterious monsters all—are the drugs we worship and fear.

When people really believed that the human body belonged to God, they concluded that there was almost nothing that physicians should be allowed to do to it (except perhaps tend to wounds to restore the body to its "natural" state).

When people really disbelieve that the human body belongs to God, they conclude that there is almost nothing that physicians should not be allowed to do to it (except perhaps destroy it with the avowed purpose of destroying it).

The religious fundamentalist thus brooks no limits in his adoration of God, creating an all-powerful deity with whose works man is forbidden to tamper. Created by and in the image of God, the human being is an infinitely valuable masterpiece which the visitors to the Divine Gallery must not touch, much less alter. For alteration is here synonymous with defacement.

Similarly, the medical fundamentalist brooks no limits in his adoration of Science, creating an all-powerful Medicine capable of endless improvements on all things biological, especially man. Created by and in the image of Medicine, the human being is a working model in the biological technician's laboratory which every "scientific worker" laboring there should attempt to alter. For alteration here is synonymous with improvement.

It is obvious that—whether because of his immoderate concept of God or because of his immoderate concept of Health—man ultimately becomes the victim of his own arrogance. It seems to me that what mankind now needs, more than anything else, is moderation and temperance in all important things; and since two of the most important things in life are religion and medicine, we need moderation and temperance with respect to God and Health. Moderation with respect to God means religious tolerance—that is, control not of the worshipper but of those who would control how he ought to worship. In the United States, the First Amendment to the Constitution, and in other free secular societies similar laws and customs, guarantee protection of the citizen from such religious molestation. Similarly, moderation with respect to Health means medical tolerance—that is, control not of the drug user but of those who would control how he ought to use drugs. But neither in the United States nor in any other modern society is the citizen protected from such medical molestation. .

In short, we must reject the images of all-powerful deities and of an all-important health-and-life. At the same time, we must retain—indeed, we must raise to much higher levels than ever before—respect for laws "higher" than man's, to symbolize that, in the court of life, a person cannot be both litigant and judge. We must thus learn to experience and exhibit genuine respect for health-and-life, to symbolize that, precisely because men and women can make life and take it, caring for it is their foremost duty. And how would people demonstrate this? Perhaps simply by re-examining and relinquishing their unshakable conviction—and their conduct based on the conviction—that care justifies coercion, and that coercion is the quintessential proof of care.

I. Pharmakos: The Scapegoat

1. THE DISCOVERY OF DRUG ADDICTION

Ever since pharmacology and psychiatry became accepted as modern medical disciplines—that is, since about the last quarter of the nineteenth century—chemists and physicians, psychologists and psychiatrists, politicians and pharmaceutical manufacturers, all have searched, in vain of course, for non-addictive drugs to relieve pain, to induce sleep, and to stimulate wakefulness. This search is based on the dual premises that addiction is a condition caused by drugs, and that some drugs are more, and others less, "addictive." This view epitomizes the confusion between the pharmacological effects of drugs and their practical uses.

When a drug deadens pain, induces sleep, or stimulates wakefulness, and when people know that there are drugs that do these things, then some persons may—depending on their personal and social circumstances and desires—develop an interest in using such drugs. Why many people habitually use such drugs, and countless other substances, need not for the moment concern us here, other than to note that the reason cannot be said to be because the drugs are "addictive." It is the other way around: we call certain drugs "addictive" because people like to use them—just as we call ether and gasoline "flammable" because they are easily ignited. It is therefore just as absurd to search for non-addictive drugs that produce euphoria as it would be to search for non-flammable liquids that are easy to ignite.

Our contemporary confusion regarding drug abuse and drug addiction is an integral part of our confusion regarding religion. Any idea or act that gives men and women a sense of what their life is about or for—that, in other words, gives their existence meaning and purpose—is, properly speaking, religious. Science, medicine, and especially health and therapy are thus admirably suited to function as quasi-religious ideas, values, and pursuits. It is necessary, therefore, to distinguish between science as science, and science as religion (sometimes called "scientism").

Since the use and avoidance of certain substances has to do with prescriptions and prohibitions, with what is legal or licit and illegal or illicit, the so-called "problem" of drug abuse or drug addiction has two aspects: religious (legal) and scientific (medical). Actually, however, since the factual or scientific aspects of this subject are negligible, the problem is, for all practical purposes, almost entirely religious or moral.[1] A simple example will amplify the nature of the distinction, and the confusion, to which I am referring.

As some persons seek or avoid alcohol and tobacco, heroin and marijuana, so others seek or avoid kosher wine and holy water. The differences between kosher wine and non-kosher wine, holy water and ordinary water, are ceremonial, not chemical. Although it would be idiotic to look for the property of kosherness in wine, or for the property of holiness in water, this does not mean that there is no such thing as kosher wine or holy water. Kosher wine is wine that is ritually clean according to Jewish law. Holy water is water blessed by a Catholic priest. This creates a certain demand for such wine and water by people who want this sort of thing; at the same time, and for precisely the same reason, such wine and water are rejected by those who do not believe in their use.

Similarly, the important differences between heroin and alcohol, or marijuana and tobacco—as far as "drug abuse" is concerned—are not chemical but ceremonial. In other words, heroin and marijuana are approached and avoided not because they are more "addictive" or more "dangerous" than alcohol and tobacco, but because they are more "holy" or "unholy"—as the case may be.

The single most important issue in coming to grips with the problem of drug use and drug avoidance is, in my opinion, the medical perspective on moral conduct. As I have shown elsewhere,[2] the psychiatric claim that personal conduct is not volitional but reflexive—in short, that human beings are not subjects but objects, not persons but organisms—was first staked out in relation to acts that were socially disturbing and could conventionally be called "mad" or "insane."

The pioneering eighteenth-century "alienists" managed the first factories for manufacturing madmen, and developed the earliest advertising campaigns for selling "insanity" by renaming badness as madness, and then offering to dispose of it. The famous nineteenth-century "neuropsychiatrists" made decisive advances in both the production and promotion of madness, establishing the "reality" of the modern concept of "mental illness": first, they progressively metaphorized disagreeable conduct and forbidden desire as disease—thus creating more and more mental diseases; second, they literalized this medical metaphor, insisting that disapproved behavior was not merely *like* a disease, but that it *was* a disease—thus confusing others, and perhaps themselves as well, regarding the differences between bodily and behavioral "abnormalities."

By the time the twentieth century was ushered in—thanks in large part to the work of Freud and the modern "psychologists" —madness was bursting through the walls of the insane asylums and was being discovered in clinics and doctors' offices, in literature and art, and in the "psychopathology of everyday life." Since the First World War, the enemies of this psychiatrization of man—in particular, religion and common sense—have lost their nerve; now they no longer even try to resist the opportunistic theories and oppressive technologies of modern "behavioral science."

Thus, by the time the contemporary American drug-abuseologists, legislators, and psychiatrists came on the scene, the contact lenses that refracted deviance as disease were so deeply embedded into the corneas of the American people that they could be pried loose only with the greatest effort; and only by leaving both the laity and the professionals so painfully wounded and temporarily blinded that they could hardly be expected to tolerate such interference with their vision, much less to impose such painful self-enlightenment on themselves.

The result was that when, in the post-Prohibition, post-Second World War, better-living-through-chemistry era, the so-called drug problem "hit" America, the phenomena it presented could be apprehended only as refracted through these irremovable contact lenses. Those who used drugs could not help themselves. Since they were the victims of their irresistible impulses, they needed others to protect them from these impulses. This made it logical and reasonable for politicians and psychiatrists to advocate "drug controls." And since none of this has "worked"—as how could it have?—the blame for it all could at least be affixed to those who sold illicit drugs: they were called "pushers" and were persecuted in the horrifying manner in which men wallowing in the conviction of their own virtuousness have always persecuted those about whose wickedness they could entertain no doubts.

Presumably some persons have always "abused" certain drugs—alcohol for millennia, opiates for centuries. However, only in the twentieth century have certain patterns of drug use been labeled as "addictions." Traditionally, the term "addiction" has meant simply a strong inclination toward certain kinds of conduct, with little or no pejorative meaning attached to it. Thus, the *Oxford English Dictionary* offers such pre-twentieth-century examples of the use of this term as being addicted "to civil affairs," "to useful reading"—and also "to bad habits." Being addicted to drugs is not among the definitions listed.

Until quite recently, then, the term "addiction" was understood to refer to a habit, good or bad as the case might be, actually more often the former. This usage saved people from the confusion into which the contemporary meaning of this term has inevitably led.

Although the term "addiction" is still often used to describe habits, usually of an undesirable sort, its meaning has become so expanded and transformed that it is now used to refer to almost any kind of illegal, immoral, or undesirable association with certain kinds of drugs. For example, a person who has smoked but a single marijuana cigarette, or even one who has not used any habit-forming or illegal drug at all, may be considered to be a drug abuser or drug addict: this is the case when a person, found to be in possession of illicit drugs, is accused by the legal and medical authorities who "examine" him of using (rather than with selling or merely carrying) these substances, and is convicted in a court of law on a charge of "drug abuse" or "drug addiction."

In short—during the past half-century, and especially during recent decades—the noun "addict" has lost its denotative meaning and reference to persons engaged in certain *habits,* and has become transformed into a stigmatizing label possessing only pejorative meaning referring to certain *persons.* The term "addict" has thus been added to our lexicon of stigmatizing labels—such as "Jew," which could mean either a person professing a certain religion or a "Christ killer" who himself should be killed; or "Negro," which could mean either a black-skinned person or a savage who ought to be kept in actual or social slavery. More specifically still, the word "addict" has been added to our psychiatric vocabulary of stigmatizing diagnoses, taking its place alongside such terms as "insane," "psychotic," "schizophrenic," and so forth.

This conceptual, cultural, and semantic transformation in the use and meaning of the term "addiction" is also reflected in its remarkably recent appearance on what psychiatrists regard as the authoritative or official lists of mental diseases or psychiatric diagnoses. The first edition of Kraepelin's classic textbook, published in 1883, lists neither drug intoxication nor drug addiction in its inventory of mental disease.[3] The second edition, published in 1887, mentions "chronic intoxications," and itemizes "alcoholism" and "morphinism," but still does not mention addiction. Four years later, in the fourth edition, "cocainism" is added to the intoxications, but addiction is still not mentioned. ("Homosexuality," however, is now added to the list.) The sixth edition, published in 1899, includes both "acute" and "chronic intoxications," noting specifically the three drugs listed previously; the same diagnoses are listed in the eighth edition, published between 1909 and 1915, with addiction still conspicuously absent.

In Bleuler's famous *Textbook of Psychiatry,* first published in 1916, "toxic psychoses" are listed among the diagnoses, but addiction is not. In the United States, the Retreat for the Insane in Hartford, Connecticut, had, in 1888, a system of classification that included "masturbation insanity" and "alcoholic insanity," but did not include intoxications or addiction. In the United States, the diagnosis of "drug addiction" became officially recognized only in 1934, when it was included for the first time among the "mental illnesses" listed in the American Psychiatric Association's *Standard Classified Nomenclature of Diseases.*[4]

The most authoritative text on the history of psychiatry, and the one most widely used today in American medical schools and psychiatric residency programs, is *A History of Psychiatry* by Gregory Zilboorg. In the index to this book, first published in 1941, there are no entries for "addiction" or "drug addiction."[5]

Ceremonial performances—such as partaking of the Holy Communion, celebrating Yom Kippur, or saluting the flag—articulate certain communal values. By participating in the ceremonial, the individual affirms his membership in the group; by refusing to participate in it, he affirms his rejection of, or withdrawal from, the group.

To understand ceremonial chemistry, we must therefore distinguish between the chemical or medical effects of drugs and the ceremonial or moral aspects of drug use. On the face of it, this is an easy enough distinction to make. If it is elusive nevertheless, it is so because—as we shall have opportunity to observe—it is a distinction we now often make at the peril of losing our valued membership in family, profession, or other group upon which our self-esteem, if not our very livelihood, depends.

The subject matter of textbooks of pharmacology is the chemical effects of various drugs on the body, especially on the human body; and, more narrowly, the use of drugs for the treatment of diseases. There is, of course, an ethical premise implicit even in this—seemingly purely medical—perspective, but this premise is so self-evident that we usually consider it unnecessary to articulate it: namely, that we regard certain drugs as "therapeutic" and seek to develop such drugs with the understanding that they are helpful to the person (patient) who uses them—and not, say, to the pathogenic microorganisms that infect or infest him, or to the cancerous cells to which he is host. A textbook of pharmacology written for pneumococci or spirochetes would not be the same as one written for human beings. The basic and yet tacit moral assumption to which I point here is that pharmacology is an applied scientific discipline—applied, that is, to the welfare of the sick patient, as that welfare is generally understood, and implemented, by the patient himself.

Nevertheless, all recent textbooks of pharmacology contain material within their pages totally inconsistent and incompatible with this aim and premise, and sharply in conflict with the ostensible intellectual task of the student or practitioner of pharmacology. I refer to the fact that all such textbooks contain a chapter on drug addiction and drug abuse.

In the fourth edition of Goodman and Gilman's *The Pharmacological Basis of Therapeutics,* Jerome H. Jaffe, a psychiatrist, defines "drug abuse" as ". . . the use, usually by self-administration, of any drug in a manner that deviates from approved medical or social patterns within a given culture."[6]

Implicitly, then, drug abuse is accepted by Jaffe, and by Goodman and Gilman—as indeed it is by nearly everyone, nearly everywhere today—as a disease whose diagnosis and treatment are the legitimate concern of the physician. But let us note carefully just what drug abuse is. Jaffe himself defines it as any deviation "from approved medical or social patterns" of drug use. We are thus immediately plunged into the innermost depths of the mythology of mental illness: for just as socially disapproved pharmacological behavior constitutes "drug abuse," and is officially recognized as an illness by a medical profession that is a licensed agency of the state, so socially disapproved sexual behavior constitutes "perversion" and is also officially recognized as an illness; and so, more generally, socially disapproved personal behavior of any kind constitutes "mental illness" which is also officially recognized as an illness—"like any other." What is particularly interesting and important about all these "illnesses"—that is, about drug abuse, sex abuse, and mental illness generally—is that few if any of the "patients" suffering from them recognize that they are sick; and that, perhaps because of this reason, these "patients" may be and frequently are "treated" against their will.[7]

As I see it, and indeed as Jaffe's own definition of it acknowledges, drug abuse is a matter of conventionality; hence, it is a subject that belongs to anthropology and sociology, religion and law, ethics and criminology—but surely not to pharmacology.

Moreover, inasmuch as drug abuse deals with disapproved or prohibited patterns of drug use, it resembles not the therapeutic use of drugs given to treat sick patients, but the toxic use of drugs given to healthy people to poison them. Some types of "drug abuse" could thus be viewed as acts of self-poisoning, standing in the same sort of logical relationship to acts of criminal poisoning as suicide' stands to homicide. But if this is so, why not also include, in textbooks of pharmacology, chapters on how to deal with those who "abuse" drugs not by poisoning themselves but by poisoning others? This, of course, seems like an absurd idea. Why? Because people who *poison other people* are criminals. What we do with them is not a problem for science or pharmacology to solve, but a decision for legislators and the courts to make. But is it any less absurd to include, in the compass of medicine or pharmacology, the problem of what to do with those persons who *poison themselves,* or who do not even harm themselves but merely violate certain social norms or legal rules?

It is clear, of course, that behind this normative or legal dimension of the drug problem there lies a biological one to which pharmacology may indeed rightfully address itself. Regardless of how a chemical substance gets into a person's body—whether through the intervention of a physician, as in ordinary medical treatment; or through self-administration, as is typically the case in drug abuse and drug addiction; or through the intervention of some malefactor, as in cases of criminal poisoning—that substance will have certain effects which we can understand better, and mitigate more successfully, if we rely on pharmacological knowledge and methods. All this is obvious. What is perhaps not so obvious is that by focusing on the chemistry of drugs we may obscure—indeed we may want to obscure—the simple fact that in some instances we deal with persons who consider themselves ill and wish to be medicated under medical control, while in others we deal with persons who do not consider themselves ill but wish to medicate themselves under their own control. The toxicological effects of drugs thus belong properly to a discussion of their other biological effects, as do the pharmacological and other measures useful for counteracting their toxicity; whereas the social and legal interventions imposed on persons called "drug abusers" or "drug addicts" have no legitimate place at all in textbooks of pharmacology.

Pharmacology, let us not forget, is the science of drug use—

that is, of the healing (therapeutic) and harming (toxic) effects of drugs. If, nevertheless, textbooks of pharmacology legitimately contain a chapter on drug abuse and drug addiction, then, by the same token, textbooks of gynecology and urology should contain a chapter on prostitution; textbooks of physiology, a chapter on perversion; textbooks of genetics, a chapter on the racial inferiority of Jews and Negroes; textbooks of mathematics, a chapter on gambling syndicates; and, of course, textbooks of astronomy, a chapter on sun worship.

The mythology of psychiatry has corrupted not only our common sense and the law but also our language and pharmacology. To be sure, as are all such corruptions and confusions, this one is not something imposed on us by conspiring or scheming psychiatrists; instead, it is simply another manifestation of the deep-seated human need for magic and religion, for ceremonial and ritual, and of the covert (unconscious) expression of this need in what we self-deceivingly think is the "science" of pharmacology.

Not until we distinguish more clearly than we now do between the chemical and ceremonial uses and effects of drugs shall we be able to begin a sensible description and a reasonable discussion of so-called problems of drug abuse and drug addiction.

It is now widely recognized and accepted that our language both reflects and shapes our experience. This sophistication has, however, had no appreciable effect on our contemporary attitudes and policies toward social problems in which the verbal shaping of the "problem" itself constitutes much or even all of the ensuing problem. We seemed to have learned little or nothing from the fact that we had no problem with drugs until we quite literally talked ourselves into having one: we declared first this and then that drug "bad" and "dangerous"; gave them nasty names like "dope" and "narcotic"; and passed laws prohibiting their use. The result: our present "problems of drug abuse and drug addiction."

The plain historical facts are that before 1914 there was no "drug problem" in the United States; nor did we have a name for it. Today there is an immense drug problem in the United States, and we have lots of names for it. Which came first: "the problem of drug abuse" or its name? It is the same as asking which came first: the chicken or the egg? All we can be sure of now is that the more chickens, the more eggs, and vice versa; and similarly, the more problems, the more names for them, and vice versa. My point is simply that our drug abuse experts, legislators, psychiatrists, and other professional guardians of our medical morals have been operating chicken hatcheries: they continue—partly by means of certain characteristic, tactical abuses of our language—to manufacture and maintain the "drug problem" they ostensibly try to solve. The following excerpts from the popular and professional press—and my comments on them—illustrate and support this contention.

From an editorial in *Science,* entitled "Death from Heroin":

> Drug abuse, which was once predominantly a disease of Harlem, is now a plague that is spreading to the suburbs. Drug use has been glamorized, while descriptions of the dreadful consequences have been muted. . . . Two relatively new methods seem promising. One is the use of methadone. A second approach is a psychiatric one, which emphasizes attitudinal changes and utilizes ex-addicts to give emotional support to those who wish to stop. . . . This nation should provide the funds to move vigorously against a spreading plague.[8]

Deaths caused by the prohibition of heroin, and especially by the contaminants added to it on the illicit market, are here falsely attributed to heroin itself; the use of heroin is called a "disease," and its spread from blacks to whites is called a "plague"; the use of methadone is considered to be a perfectly legitimate type of medical treatment for the heroin habit, while no mention is made of the fact that the use of heroin originated as a treatment for the morphine habit. Furthermore, psychiatric interventions with persons stigmatized as "drug abusers" and "drug addicts" are here misrepresented as "help" which the "patients" want in order to stop taking illegal drugs, whereas it is actually something imposed on them by law by those who want them to stop this habit; and the policies of psychiatrically harassing persons who take illegal drugs, and of using tax monies to supply them with legal drugs (such as methadone), are accepted unquestioningly and uncritically as medically indicated and morally justified.

From a report in the *Syracuse Herald-Journal* entitled "New Drug Offers Hope: May Immunize Heroin Addicts":

> The drug is EN-1639A from laboratories in Garden City, N.Y. Industry sources confirmed the firm is close to clinical testing, the last step before marketing of a new drug. . . . EN-1639A has already been tested on some human subjects at the federal drug rehabilitation and addiction center at Lexington, Ky. Officials there believe the new drug could wipe out addiction the way vaccines have eliminated smallpox.[9]

This is an illustration of some of the consequences of mistaking metaphor for the thing metaphorized. Addiction is no longer *like* a plague; it *is* a plague. A drug compulsorily administered to addicts is no longer *like* a vaccine; it *is* a vaccine.

From a report in *The New York Times* entitled "Amphetamines Used by a Physician to Lift Moods of Famous Patients":

> For many years Dr. Max Jacobson, a 72-year old general practitioner in New York, has been injecting amphetamine—the powerful stimulant the drug culture calls "speed"—into the veins of dozens of the country's most celebrated artists, writers, politicians, and jet-setters. . . . Dr. Jacobson is the best known of a small number of New York doctors who specialize in prescribing and administering amphetamines not to treat disease but to boost the mood of healthy patients. Far from the typical picture of rag-tag youths dosing themselves with illegally obtained drugs, the story of Dr. Jacobson and his patients is one of wealthy and famous adults depending on a licensed physician for their completely legal injections. . . . The most famous of the doctor's patients were President and Mrs. Kennedy. . . . In 1961, for example, he went with the President to Vienna for the summit meeting with Khrushchev and, Dr. Jacobson said in an interview, gave the President injections there. . . . Once, when Dr. Jacobson was in the audience for the Boston try-out of Mr. [Alan Jay] Lerner's "On a Clear Day," he turned to Mrs. Burton Lane, the wife of the musical's composer, and made a boast that many persons said he often makes. As Mrs. Lane recalled it, Dr. Jacobson pointed to his tie clip, a PT-109 insignia, and said, "Do you know where I got this? I worked with the Kennedys. I travelled with the Kennedys. I treated the Kennedys. Jack Kennedy. Jacqueline Kennedy. They never could have made it without me.

They gave me this in gratitude." . . . Jacqueline Kennedy Onassis confirmed through a spokesman that she had been treated by Dr. Jacobson but declined to elaborate.[10]

The medicalization of the English language has here progressed so far that we have not only "sick patients" but also "healthy patients"; and that we have "treatments" not only for making sick persons better but also for making healthy persons more energetic. To be sure, these distinctions apply only to the powerful and the wealthy: when they take psychoactive drugs, they are still respected political leaders who, in their spare time, wage war on drug abuse; when the powerless and the poor take the same drugs, they are "dope fiends" bent on destroying the nation. The ancient Latin adage *Quod licet Jovi, non licet bovi* ("What is permitted to Jove is not permitted to the cow") is, perhaps, more relevant to our understanding of the uses of licit and illicit drugs than all the chemical facts and fantasies about drug abuse assembled in textbooks of pharmacology and psychiatry.

In an address at the annual legislative dinner of the Empire State Chamber of Commerce, Governor Nelson Rockefeller declares: "We, the citizens, are imprisoned by pushers. I want to put the pushers in prison so we can come out, ladies and gentlemen."[11]

Glester Hinds, the head of Harlem's People's Civic and Welfare Association, commenting on Governor Rockefeller's proposal for mandatory life sentences without parole for heroin pushers, states: "I don't think the Governor went far enough. It should be included in his bill as capital punishment because these murderers need to be gotten rid of completely."[12]

Dr. George W. McMurray, pastor of the Mother African Methodist Episcopal Zion Church, commends Rockefeller for his "forthright stand against addiction," which he calls a "subtle form of genocidal execution."[13]

William F. Buckley, in a column on Governor Rockefeller's proposals for dealing with heroin pushers, writes: "One shrinks from the medieval concern to design modes of death particularly appropriate to the crime of the offender. . . . But it is not, I should think, inappropriate to suggest that a condign means of ridding the world of convicted heroin pushers is to prescribe an overdose. It happens that it is a humane way of dying, if one defines humane as relatively painless. And, of course, there is a rabbinical satisfaction in the idea that the pusher should leave this world in such circumstances as he has caused others to leave it. . . ."[14]

Here we are told, by a variety of authorities, that citizens are imprisoned by pushers, when, in fact, the citizens' safety is imperiled by legislators and politicians who, by prohibiting the sale and use of heroin, create the crimes associated with the illegal market in it; that pushers are "murderers" who should be executed, when, in fact, pushers commit no harm, much less murder, and when there is no death penalty in New York State even for first-degree murder; that "addiction is a form of genocidal execution," when, in fact, it is an expression of self-determination; and that heroin pushers are murderers who should be killed by giving them an overdose of heroin, again advocating the death sentence for metaphorical murderers even though there is no such sentence for literal murderers.

makes sense & valid pt

not TRUE inaccurate

From an address by Rep. James M. Hanley (D.-N.Y.) before the Baldwinsville, N.Y., Chamber of Commerce:

> Rep. Hanley called the 60,000 known drug addicts in the U.S. only "the visible portion of the iceberg," and expressed concern over unknown present and potential addicts, asking "how many vermin are infesting our high schools and colleges," pushing this junk on our unwary youth?[15]

Rep. Hanley here uses the same metaphor for condemning persons who use or sell illegal drugs that the Nazis used to justify murdering Jews by poisoned gas—namely, that the persecuted persons are not human beings but "vermin."

From a Letter to the Editor of *The New York Times* by Steven Jonas, M.D., Assistant Professor of Community Medicine at the State University of New York, Stony Brook, Long Island:

> Governor Rockefeller's new proposal for dealing with the drug problem by attacking sellers [by imposing mandatory life sentences

he tries to parallel "pushers" & legislators as Jews & Nazi's — yet drug dealers are not innocent by any means much less victims.

on those who sell "dangerous drugs"] are strongly supported by epidemiological theory. Heroin addiction in particular is much like a communicable disease, even though noninfectious. There are a host, man, an agent, heroin, and identifiable environmental factors, just like there are in infectious communicable diseases. Furthermore, there is a vector, or carrier, or the agent, the pusher (and dealer), who may or may not be infected himself. Thus heroin addiction is similar in many ways to diseases such as malaria with its identifiable vector, the mosquito.[16]

A physician who is a professor in a medical school here asserts that heroin addiction is like malaria, that heroin is like a parasite, and that the person who sells heroin is like a mosquito. The verminization of the human being, begun by the Health Ministry of National Socialist Germany, is thus continued—without any public recognition that it is—through the American war on "drug abuse."

Clearly, the differences between the past and the present—the traditional moral and the modern medical—uses of the term "addict" could hardly be greater. In the first case, we have a *description—a name—*not entirely value-free, to be sure, but identifying mainly a particular habit on the part of the person to whom it is applied. In the second case, we have an *ascription—an epithet—*not entirely fact-free, to be sure (unless it is used mistakenly or mendaciously), but identifying mainly a particular *judgment* on the part of the person making it. In its descriptive sense, the term "addiction" tells us something about what the "addict" does *to himself;* in its ascriptive sense, it tells us something about what those making the judgment plan to do *to him.*

I have made this same sort of distinction—between fact and value, description and ascription, self-definition and definition by others—in several of my previous works: In particular, I have tried to show that there are not only two different psychiatries, voluntary and involuntary—but that they are antagonistic to one another; and I have tried to demonstrate that to confuse and combine these two can lead only to mystification for the psychiatrists and misfortune for the so-called patients.[17] Nowhere could these distinctions be more obvious than in the area of so-called drug abuse and drug addiction: for the facts here, quite simply, are that some people want to take some drugs which some others do not want them to take. The drug users—called "drug abusers" or "drug addicts" by the authorities—regard their drugs as their allies, and those who try to deprive them of the drugs as their adversaries; whereas the politicians, psychiatrists, and ex-addicts—who call themselves "experts on drug abuse and drug addiction"—regard the prohibited drugs as their enemies, the persons who use them as their "patients," and their own coercive interventions as "treatments."

It seems to me that a great deal of current thinking and writing about addiction is vitiated—is made meaningless, misleading, and mischievous—by a persistent failure or refusal to make the distinctions outlined above. Assertions are made, rejoinders are offered, and the whole subject is hotly debated, without bothering to scrutinize what is meant by the terms "addict" and "addiction." One reason for all this is that it is much easier to examine the chemical effects of a drug a person uses than the social effects of a ceremony he performs.

It requires intelligence to understand the chemistry of a drug one takes, but it requires courage to understand the ceremony one performs; and while it requires intelligence to understand the chemistry of a drug others take, it requires both courage and tolerance to understand the ceremony they perform. Intelligence, courage, and tolerance are all in short supply, decreasing in that order. So long as that remains the human condition, the so-called human sciences will continue to lag far behind the natural sciences.

To understand holy water, we must of course examine priests and parishioners, not water; and to understand abused and addictive drugs, we must examine doctors and addicts, politicians and populations, not drugs. Clearly, some situations are more favorable for such an enterprise than others. One could not very well study holy water in medieval Italy or Spain, especially if one was, and hoped to remain, a good Catholic. In the same way, one cannot very well study opium and heroin, or marijuana and methadone, in the U.S.A. or U.S.S.R., especially if one is, and hopes to remain, a loyal physician whose duty is to help combat the "plague" of drug abuse and drug addiction.

Social ceremonies serve to unite individuals in groups. They often perform this function well, albeit at a high cost to certain individuals in the system, or to certain values cherished by the group. Because the scrutiny of ceremonials tends to weaken their cohesive powers, it is perceived as a threat to the group. Herein lies the basic limitation to the feasibility and influence of the analysis of ritual, whether magical or medical.

2. THE SCAPEGOAT AS DRUG AND THE DRUG AS SCAPEGOAT

Thousands of years ago—in times we are fond of calling "primitive" (since this renders us "modern" without having to exert ourselves further to earn this qualification)—religion and medicine were a united and undifferentiated enterprise; and both were closely allied with government and politics—all being concerned with maintaining the integrity of the community and of the individuals who were its members. How did ancient societies and their priest-physicians protect people from plagues and famines, from the perils of impending military encounters, and from all the other calamities that threaten persons and peoples? They did so, in general, by performing certain religious ceremonies.

In ancient Greece (as elsewhere), one of these ceremonies consisted of human sacrifice. The selection, naming, special treatment, and finally the ritualized destruction of the scapegoat was the most important and most potent "therapeutic" intervention known to "primitive" man. In ancient Greece, the person sacrificed as a scapegoat was called the *pharmakos*. The root of modern terms such as pharmacology and pharmacopeia is therefore not "medicine," "drug," and "poison," as most dictionaries erroneously state, but "scapegoat"! To be sure, after the practice of human sacrifice was abandoned in Greece, probably around the sixth century B.C., the word did come to mean "medicine," "drug," and "poison." Interestingly, in modern Albanian *pharmak* still means only "poison."

The "modern" reader might be tempted to shrug off all this as etymological curiosity. The magic in which his ancestors believed he considers "nonsense." He doesn't believe in magic. He "believes" only in facts, in science, in medicine. Insofar as this critical characterization of the modern mind is accurate, it shows us starkly two things: first, that just as human anatomy and physiology have changed little if at all during the past, say, three thousand years, so social organizations and the principles of social control have also changed little if at all; and second, that, in some ways at least, modern man may be more "primitive" than was ancient man. When the ancients saw a scapegoat, they could at least recognize him for what he was: a *pharmakos,* a human sacrifice. When modern man sees one, he does not, or refuses to, recognize him for what he is; instead, he looks for "scientific" explanations—to explain away the obvious. Thus, to the modern mind, the witches were mentally sick women; the Jews in Nazi Germany were the victims of a mass psychosis; involuntary mental patients are sick people unaware of their own need for treatment; and so on. I submit, and will try to show, that among the long list of scapegoats which the insatiable human appetite for *pharmakoi* seems to demand, some of the most important today are certain substances—called "dangerous drugs," "narcotics," or "dope"; certain entrepreneurs—called "pushers" or "drug traffickers"; and certain persons who use certain prohibited substances—called "drug addicts," "drug abusers," or "drug-dependent persons." This pseudoscientific and pseudomedical language is both the cause and the result of the shocking modern insensibility concerning scapegoating, and insensitivity toward scapegoats. Civilized man, in contrast to his primitive forebear, "knows" that opium is a dangerous narcotic; that people who sell it are evil individuals, properly analogized with, and treated as, murderers; and that persons who use it are at once sick and sinful, and should be "treated" against their will for their own good—in short, he "knows" that none of them is a scapegoat. Thus, an advertisement for the new 1973 New York State drug law concludes with this revealing plea and promise: "Protect the addicts from themselves and help make New York a better place to live."[1]

The ancient Greeks would have recognized the situation to which this law refers, and of which it is itself an important part, as having to do with *pharmakoi,* rather than with pharmacology. We don't. The fact that we don't is a measure of man's irrepressible inhumanity to man, expressed through his unappeasable appetite for human sacrifice. I shall try to show how this appetite is now satisfied through our belief in pharmacomythology and through its characteristic rituals of ceremonial chemistry. To follow my argument, it will be necessary to suspend our faith in conventional wisdom, especially as that wisdom now defines and sees the Church, the State, and Medicine.

The First Amendment to the Constitution of the United States decrees a separation between Church and State, thus implying that they are separate and separable institutions. In a similar way, modern societies distinguish sharply between religion and medicine, clergymen and physicians, implying that the priestly and medical enterprises and institutions are separate and separable. Within certain—quite narrow—limits, and for certain—quite discrete—purposes, it is indeed possible and desirable to distinguish religion from medicine, and each from government. However, these distinctions, and the habits of language and mind that they engender, have made us lose sight of some very old, very simple, and very profound truths: in particular, that the most important business of every society is the regulation of the behavior of its members; that there was, in the ancient world, no separation between the roles of priest and physician; and that, in the modern world also, Church, Medicine, and State continue to collaborate in maintaining social order by regulating personal conduct.

The fundamental concept with respect to social control is, of course, "law," which was formerly "rabbinical," "canonical," and "ecclesiastic"—as well as "secular," "political," or "legal"; and which is now ostensibly wholly "secular" or "legal"—while it is actually also "religious" and "political," and most importantly "medical" and "psychiatric." It is impressive testimony to our powers of self-deception that we believe we can expand our civil liberties by opposing threats to it from politicians, while at the same time inviting and embracing threats to it from physicians and psychiatrists.

Illustrative of these threats to our liberties, and of the essential unity of religious, medical, and legal concepts and sanctions in the laws that threaten them, are the new New York State drug laws which became effective on September 1, 1973. In large—nearly full-page—newspaper advertisements warning people: "Don't Get Caught Holding the Bag," the purpose of the new laws is explained as follows: "To deter people from the unlawful sale or possession of illegal drugs and to rehabilitate those people who are, or are in

imminent danger of becoming, dependent on these drugs."² The
idea of "rehabilitating" persons from the "imminent danger of becoming dependent" on drugs which the government of the State
of New York does not want them to use is, of course, essentially
religious, with respect to both the offense and the sanctions for it.

The amalgamation of medicine, psychiatry, and law, implicit in
all such laws, is made fully explicit in the advertisement by the
names of the new laws—which are: "Public Health Law: Article
33; Mental Hygiene Law: Article 81; Penal Law: Article 220."
We further learn that "the drug laws provide a schedule of crimes
. . . and related penalties." "Addicts" are then urged to get "treatment": "Besides enforcing the law, the State is spending money
for drug abuse treatment. . . . A treatment program is available
24 hours a day. All you have to do is call!"³

The contents of these laws—that is, the behaviors proscribed
and the penalties prescribed for them—illustrate, finally, the combined magical, medical, and political character of such legislation.
The penalty for the unlawful possession of two ounces or more of
"any narcotic substance" is "15 years to life imprisonment";
for the unlawful possession of one ounce or more of marijuana,
it is one to fifteen years of imprisonment; and for the unlawful
possession of five milligrams or more of LSD, it is one year to life
imprisonment.

To understand why some people take certain substances, and
why others declare these substances "unlawful" and savagely punish those who take them, we must begin at the beginning, with the
basic principles of social congregation and social control.

In her classic study of Greek religion, Jane Ellen Harrison describes what she considers to be a fundamental law of social organization in general, and of religious ritual in particular—namely,
"the conservation and promotion of life."⁴ This protection of the
life of both the individual and the community is achieved "in
two ways, one negative, one positive, by the riddance of whatever
is conceived to be hostile, and by the enhancement of whatever
is conceived of as favorable to life."⁵

In order that he may live, writes Harrison, "primitive man
has before him the old dual task to get rid of evil, and secure good.

Evil is to him of course mainly hunger and barrenness. Good is food and fertility. The Hebrew word for 'good' meant originally good to eat."[6] Individuals and societies thus seek to include that which they consider good, and to exclude that which they consider evil. This principle may also be inverted: individuals or groups may, and often do, promote or prohibit certain substances to justify defining them as good or bad. The ritual thus symbolizes and defines the character of the substance that is ceremonially sought or avoided, and the belief about the goodness or badness of the substance in turn supports the ritual. This explains the social stability of such beliefs and rituals and their relative immunity to "rational" or "scientific" arguments seeking to alter them. It also explains why some individuals and groups are as deeply committed to the (ritual) use of certain substances—such as alcohol or opium, beef or pork—as others are to their (ritual) avoidance.

The ceremonial of the scapegoat is surely one of the most important instances and prototypes of all riddance rituals. In Greece during the first century A.D., the scapegoat was not killed but only ritually expelled. The ceremony was described by Plutarch (c. 46–120), who, as chief magistrate of his native town, himself performed the ceremony, playing the role, of course, of the scapegoater. Harrison describes the ceremony as follows: "The little township of Chaeronea in Boeotia, Plutarch's birthplace, saw enacted year by year a strange and very ancient ceremonial. It was called 'The Driving out of the Famine.' A household slave was driven out of doors with rods of *agnus castus,* a willow-like plant, and over him were pronounced the words, 'Out with Famine, in with Health and Wealth.' "[7]

While this was merely a mock sacrifice of the scapegoat, there were actual scapegoat sacrifices in Greece, both before Plutarch's time and after it. At one time, Frazer tells us, the Athenians maintained "a number of degraded and useless beings at public expense; and when any calamity . . . befell the city, they sacrificed two of these outcast scapegoats."[8] Moreover, such sacrifices were not confined to extraordinary occasions but were regular religious ceremonials. Every year, Frazer writes, "at the festival of the Thargelia in May, two victims, one for the men and one for the women, were led out of Athens and stoned to death. The city of Abdera in Thrace was publicly purified once a year, and one of the burghers, set apart for the purpose, was stoned to death as a scapegoat or vicarious sacrifice for the life of all the others. . . ."[9]

As I have mentioned earlier, the Greek name for persons so sacrificed was *pharmakoi*. John Cuthbert Lawson's account of this ritual human sacrifice is instructive in this connection: "If calamity overtook the city through divine wrath, whether it were famine or pestilence or any other bane, a *pharmakos* was led out to an appointed place for sacrifice. Cheese, barley-cake, and dried figs were given to him. He was smitten seven times on the privy parts with squills and wild figs and other wild plants; and finally he was burnt with fire upon fuel collected from wild trees, and the ashes were scattered to the winds and the sea."[10]

This sort of explicit destruction of human scapegoats is distasteful to the more "civilized" or "modern" mentality, which prefers to disguise its ceremonials of scapegoating. For example, Gilbert Murray observes: "The memory of a time when human beings had been deliberately slaughtered as a way of pleasing God runs through the literature of the fifth century as of something far-off, romantic, horrible. We may compare it to our own memories of the burning of heretics and witches, deeds which we know to have been done quite lately, by men very like ourselves, and yet deeds which we can scarcely conceive as psychologically possible to any sane being. In just the same way, to the earliest of the great Athenians, Aeschylus, the sacrifice of Iphigenia is something monstrous, beyond understanding. The man who did it must have been mad. To Euripides such acts are generally connected with a study of the worst possibilities of the savage mob, or of scheming kings led by malignant and half-insane priests."[11]

It is significant, then, how deeply pervasive the human passion is not only for victimizing scapegoats but also for trying to conceal this passion by attributing it to madness.

According to Murray, the word *pharmakos* "means literally 'human medicines' or 'scapegoats.' "[12] Martin Nilsson offers a similar but even more telling interpretation of it. The *pharmakoi*, he asserts, were "like a sponge with which one dries a table [who] when they have absorbed all the impurity, are entirely destroyed so that this impurity shall be altogether removed with them; they are thrown away, burnt up, cast into the sea. And that is why this 'sacrifice,' so-called, need not, like others, be without blemish or defect. A dog may be used, which was otherwise never sacrificed, or a condemned criminal. He was called *pharmakos*, 'remedy,' *peripsema*, 'off-scouring,' or *katharmada*, 'that which is wiped off'; this last word in particular clearly shows the meaning of the rite. We can understand how these words came to mean 'scum' and became the worst terms of abuse in the Greek language. A victim of this nature is a scapegoat upon which all evil is loaded, but which, instead of being let loose and driven into the desert, is completely destroyed, together with its evil burden."[13]

The similarities between this imagery and that conjured up by the burning of heretics, witches, Jews, and prohibited books and drugs are arresting and significant. And so are also the similarities between the later mitigated ceremonials of the *pharmakos* and the contemporary mitigated ceremonial incarcerations, rather than incinerations, of madmen and drug abusers.

For an account of a modified scapegoat ceremonial, Murray refers to Ister, a third-century historian, who gave this account of the ritual: "Two persons, one for the men of the city, one for the women, were led out as though to execution. They wore necklaces, one of white figs, the other of black. They seem to have been solemnly presented with cake and figs, and then scourged and pelted out of the city. . . . At the end, the *pharmakoi* were supposed to be dead and their ashes were thrown into the sea. The ceremony was an 'imitation,' says Ister, of a stoning to death."[14]

Murray is not impressed by this disclaimer, and cites instances of human sacrifice which contradict Ister. He is, indeed, fully aware of the depth of the human passion for scapegoating, so easily mobilized in times of public anguish and distress. "As a matter of fact," adds Murray, "it is just on occasions like this that human sacrifices have most tended to occur: in a disorganized army or a rabble full of fear, egged on by some fanatical priest or prophet.

There were bloody doings in Rome when the fear of Hannibal was strong, judicial murders of vestal virgins, burying alive of 'Gallus et Galla, Graecus et Graeca' in the Forum Boarium."[15]

By the early 1960s, a generation after triumphing over all their enemies in the Second World War, the American people were also full of fears, and were egged on by fanatical priests of drug-abuseology. The result was the invention of a new imagery of pollution—by drugs, drug pushers, and drug addicts; and of a correspondingly new category of *pharmakoi*—whose burden of evil is, literally, pharmacological.

To be sure, there is an important difference between the ancient Greek *pharmakos* and the modern American pharmacological scapegoat. The former, an expendable person, was an object or thing: he or she was an effigy or symbol—the scapegoat—in a purification ceremony. The latter (when an individual rather than a drug), although still an expendable person, is both object and subject, thing and agent: he or she is an effigy or symbol—the scapegoat—in a purification ceremony; and also a participant—the addict or pusher—in a counter-ceremony celebrating a substance tabooed by society's dominant ethic.

Many of the most dramatic moments of history, both biblical and secular, have to do with *pharmakoi*. According to Paton, Adam and Eve were *pharmakoi*,[16] an interpretation that would make God the first scapegoater. Certainly, the legend is consistent with God's need to purify His Garden, polluted by Man's ingestion of a forbidden substance. All men and women are thus scapegoats. When they reject this role, they often do so by becoming scapegoaters.

Abraham's near-sacrifice of his son transforms Isaac into still another *pharmakos,* and supports the imagery of the Jewish God as a scapegoater. The self-definition of the Jews as God's Chosen People may thus be viewed as their attempt to escape from the role of scapegoat by casting all non-Jews into that role through their implicit status as God's stepchildren or castoffs.

That the central figure in the Christian religions is a *pharmakos* is obvious. Christ, moreover, was a great healer even while "alive." Resurrected as a deity, He is truly the Christian *panacea,* the cure-all for all ills, a function previously discharged, as we have seen, through the ceremonial killing of the *pharmakos*.

Thus we come full circle: from *pharmakoi to pharmacology*; from cure-alls through human sacrifice to cure-alls through chemistry; and to the sacrifice of pharmacological *pharmakoi*—through whose expulsion Man, the god of chemistry, seeks to purify his polluted earthly Garden.

3. MEDICINE: THE FAITH
OF THE FAITHLESS

I have argued that the sacrificial principle of purgation by scapegoat is fundamental to the maintenance of human societies. Inasmuch as this is, historically speaking, a religious concept and
ceremony—as exemplified by the celebration of the Jewish Yom
Kippur and by the Christian Holy Communion—we must inquire
into the fate of this principle under conditions no longer favorable
to religious institutions and practices, such as prevail in the modern
world. Perhaps more than anyone else, Kenneth Burke has appreciated and warned that "the sacrificial principle of victimage ('the
scapegoat') is intrinsic to human congregation";[1] and has wisely
suggested that our task, as students of human behavior and as
humanists, is "not how the sacrificial motives revealed in the
institutions of magic and religion might be eliminated in a scientific
culture, but [to show] what new forms they take."[2]

I have noted elsewhere that, as medical values have replaced
religious values, medical rituals have taken the place of religious
rituals.[3] The new principle is: whatever promotes health—good
food, good drugs, good heredity, good habits—must be incorporated
or cultivated; whatever promotes illness—poisons, microbes, tainted
heredity, bad habits—must be eliminated or discouraged. Accordingly, I have suggested that we regard the entire mental health
movement as a gigantic pseudomedical ritual: that which is considered good is defined as mentally healthy and is embraced; that
which is considered bad is defined as mentally sick and is repudiated. The perspective on drug abuse and drug addiction which
I develop in this book is actually a special instance—at the present
time, economically and socially the most important instance—of
this ceremonial function of the mental health movement.

It is a remarkable fact—and a revealing one, as we shall see—
that the ritual character of our so-called drug problem and the
attempts to control it (which, of course, are two faces of the same
coin) is so consistently ignored or overlooked.

"Alcohol and Christianity," said Nietzsche, are "the two great

European narcotics." "Religion is the opium of the people," added Marx. Nearly everyone knows these aphorisms. But, clearly, hardly anyone takes them seriously. It is essential that we understand why this is so.

To make life meaningful and livable, people have always depended on certain beliefs and practices, which used to be called religions; they have also always depended on certain substances whose use formed an integral part of their religious practices.

These facts have not changed. But our perspective on them, and the vocabulary we use to describe and to try to understand them, have changed. Modern man either turns his back on religion (*qua* religion), or is consciously, if not proudly, hostile to it. In the Communist world, the anti-religious mentality is deliberately cultivated because religion is viewed as inimical to the dialectical-materialist principles on which the state ostensibly rests and which it uses to justify its policies; whereas in the so-called "free world," the anti-religious mentality is unwittingly encouraged because religion is viewed as inimical to the rational-scientific principles on which the economy and industry of the state rest and which the government uses to justify its domestic, and especially its health and welfare, policies.

Man, however, cannot live without religion. The objects of his faith and his religious practices have thus become transformed and renamed: into the worship of the Communist state, in the East; and into the worship of science and the "general welfare," in the West.

All this has often been remarked and written about. What has been surprisingly neglected and unappreciated is a cultural change running parallel with this worldwide anti-religious sentiment and indeed forming an integral part of it—namely, the sentiment and movement against the ceremonial use of drugs, and especially against the personal use of certain mood-affecting drugs condemned by physicians and criminalized by politicians. However, since most people cannot live without drugs any more than they can without religion, these veritable crusades against ceremonial drugs have generated compensatory drives to provide people with what appears so indispensable for their spiritual existence.

Having successfully deprived vast numbers of persons of the legitimate use of drugs to which they had been accustomed (or in whose use they have more recently become interested), the governments of the leading nations of the world now satisfy the unquenchable craving of their people for ceremonial drugs in one, or several, of these three ways: first, by legitimizing certain drugs by defining them as not drugs at all, and by encouraging their consumption—for example, alcohol and tobacco in the U.S. and the U.S.S.R.; second, by tacitly fostering an illicit trade in prohibited drugs—for example, heroin and marijuana in the U.S.; and third, by aggressively promoting the use, through medical prescriptions, of certain types of new (non-traditional) mood-affecting drugs— for example, synthetic psychopharmacologicals throughout the civilized world.

If it is true that the phenomena we now call drug addiction and drug abuse constitute certain kinds of ceremonial behaviors, then it follows that they can be understood only in terms appropriate to the analysis of ceremonial, as against technical, performances. I am here using the terms "ceremony" and "ceremonial" in their customary sense, meaning action, behavior, or conduct governed by prescribed rules, usually of a traditional sort. The rules may be prescribed by an institution, such as a church, court, army, or school, or by social expectations handed down through culture and suffused through the whole community. Thus, the synonyms of ceremonial are conventional, religious, ritual, and symbolic; and its antonyms are personal, scientific, technical, and idiosyncratic. A few examples will illustrate some aspects of this distinction most relevant to my subsequent argument.

To survive we must eat certain kinds of foods, but the choice of what we actually eat is determined more by social ceremony than by physiological necessity. For example, the flesh of cats and dogs would sustain us as well as does the flesh of hogs and cattle; we eat the latter and not the former for reasons of convention, not of biology. Similarly, when Jews avoid pork, Hindus beef, and vegetarians the meat of all animals, they do so for reasons that are properly called ceremonial.

We need to experience communion with our fellow human beings—and sometimes with the forces we attribute to nature, the universe, or a godhead—and to satisfy this need we use, among other things, certain substances that affect our feelings and behavior. Sometimes some of these substances are called "drugs," and their effects on individuals and groups are said to be "mental."

Actually, the effects of so-called psychoactive drugs—as opposed to the effects of antibiotics, diuretics, and many other types of pharmacological agents—are determined partly by their chemical composition and partly by the expectations of those who use them. It is these expectations—especially with respect to the substance to which they are directed, that is, whether toward alcohol, marijuana, opium, or cocaine—that vary from culture to culture and from time to time. And it is precisely these expectations which, because they constitute an integral part of a culture—just as its language or religion does—cannot be easily changed, especially by what those who hold them consider to be alien or hostile interests. Indeed, such assaults against them often serve only to strengthen the communal solidarity and inflame the religious zeal of the group: we see—and we generally understand and accept—this phenomenon for what it is in cases of religious persecutions and wars of colonial conquest; but we seem quite blind to it—and hence we neither understand nor accept it—when we encounter this same phenomenon in relation to persecutions for ceremonial drug use. The American experience with Prohibition was an astonishing illustration of this very phenomenon: a deeply entrenched, tradition-sanctioned pattern of drug use was abruptly prohibited by law. The result was that the interest in alcohol, suddenly driven · underground, increased; Prohibition greatly strengthened, rather than weakened, the ceremonial aspects of drinking. The speakeasy became a veritable secret church or temple; and the American vocabulary having to do with drink, drinking places, and drunkenness expanded remarkably.[4]

In the distant past—when culture was a carrier of tradition rather

than, as it is in many modern societies, a court for the adjudica-
tion of social and personal conflicts—people understood ritual behavior better than they do now. The decline not only of religious
and patriotic ceremonies—but also of good manners testifies, I
think, to this observation. Perhaps because, of all the major modern
nations, the United States is the least tradition-bound, Americans
are most prone to misapprehend and misinterpret ritual as something else: the result is that we mistake magic for medicine, and
confuse ceremonial effect with chemical cause.

The analysis of ritual symbolism—in our present case, the ritual
symbolism associated with using and avoiding, promoting and
prohibiting, various substances—requires that certain conditions for
it be fulfilled, foremost among them, according to Mary Douglas,
that "we recognize ritual as an attempt to create and maintain a
particular culture, a particular set of assumptions by which experience is controlled."[5] Obviously, we cannot recognize the ritual
symbolism of the pretrial psychiatric examination of a person accused of assassinating a President so long as we believe that there
is an illness called "mental illness" which can "make" a person
kill Presidents. In this particular case, our assumptions are those
of contemporary psychiatry, and we interpret our rituals as applications of the "science of psychiatry" to the "administration of
the criminal law." Similarly, we cannot recognize the ritual symbolism of our medical, psychiatric, and political pronouncements
and practices concerning, for example, the uses of marijuana and
tobacco so long as we believe that these declarations are not ritual
acts directed toward maintaining our culture, but are rather medical acts directed toward maintaining the physical and mental health
of our citizens.

The need to "create and maintain a particular culture," and the
effort to satisfy this need, apply all the way from the largest col-
lectives down to a single individual. As a general rule, the character and significance of such ritual symbolism are repressed, remain
unrecognized, until one compares his own everyday customs
with respect to eating, drinking, speaking, drug taking, and
so forth with those of others—which is what anthropologists often
do; or until one confronts his own "bad" habits and tries to change

them—which is what persons in psychotherapy often do or ought to do. I list a few examples below by way of illustration.

We eat chicken and beef and, because we do, feel superior to people who do not. And we do not eat cats and dogs and, because we do not, feel superior to those who do. Such examples could, of course, be multiplied a thousandfold.[6] Each teaches the same lesson: namely, that our culturally shared customs and habits are God-given, natural, scientific, and healthy—whereas those of others are heretical, unnatural, irrational, and unhealthy.

One of the most interesting examples of our propensity to believe that our rituals are a matter not of magic but of medicine, that they serve the aims not of ceremony but of hygiene, is our attitude toward our own saliva. While saliva remains in the mouth, we regard it as a part of our own body: it is clean and we swallow it as a matter of course. But once outside of the mouth, we no longer regard saliva as a part of our body: now called "sputum," it is dirty, and we are revolted at the mere thought of taking it back into our mouth, much less swallowing it. The same sort of imagery and idea applies to masticated food in our mouth as against the same material spit out, or, still worse, expelled from the stomach.

The point to remember here is that ceremony is not chemistry. It would be pointless for a physician to argue that saliva spit out on a clean handkerchief is identical to saliva in the mouth, and that therefore we should not feel repelled by it or opposed to swallowing it. We are repelled by such sputum not because it is dirty, but the other way around: we regard it as dirty in order to maintain our justification for feeling repelled by it! It is the same way with opium. It would be pointless for a pharmacologist to argue that smoking opium is less harmful for the human organism than smoking tobacco, and that therefore we should not prohibit it. We are repelled by the opium habit not because it is harmful, but the other way around: we regard it as harmful in order to maintain our justification for prohibiting it.

In the secular-scientific perspective of our age, we try to see all kinds of religious rituals as "rational" for the circumstances in which they originated, rather than as genuinely or truly religious.

In this view, which Douglas skillfully satirizes, "the importance of incense is not that it symbolizes the ascending smoke of sacrifice, but it is a means of making tolerable the smells of unwashed humanity. Jewish and Islamic avoidance of pork is explained as due to the dangers of eating pig in hot climates."[7] Such reinterpretations show the limitless powers of the human mind to see what it wants to see. "Even if some of Moses's dietary rules were hygienically beneficial," concludes Douglas, "it is a pity to treat him as an enlightened public health administrator rather than as a spiritual leader."[8]

The issue before us now, of course, is a reversal of these roles: we treat spiritual leaders as if they were public health administrators! We thus pay homage, and huge salaries as well, to psychiatrists and other mental health workers to combat the "plague" of drug addiction, as if they were bona fide physicians—when actually they are priests clothed in the mantle of medicine, the raiment appropriate for the priesthood of the scientific age.

Furthermore, the very concepts of clean and dirty (unclean) are, originally, religious concepts. The fact that we now use the same words with medical meanings attached to them both obscures and clarifies the distinction between medicine and magic. For example, the Jewish dietary laws, as set forth in Leviticus and Deuteronomy, specify long lists of foods that may be eaten, called "clean," and that may not be eaten, called "unclean" or "abominable things."[9] Douglas devotes a whole chapter to refuting the countless modern attempts to give some sort of functional, "rational" interpretation to these rules, including the interpretation that these rules were intended as moral exercises for inculcating self-control in the Jews; and to showing that all these attempts are grounded in the desire to rob these rules of their symbolic significance as definers of what is "clean" and hence acceptable to God, and what is "unclean" and hence unacceptable to Him.[10] To be clean, to be whole, and to be holy are, in this religious-symbolic sense, closely related notions. Much of Leviticus is devoted to enumerating the criteria of the physical intactness required of persons going to the temple and of the animals offered for sacrifice: "And the Lord said to Moses, 'Say to Aaron, None of your descendants throughout their generations who has a blemish shall draw near, a man blind or lame, or one who has a mutilated face or limb too long, or a man who has an injured foot or an injured hand, or a hunchback, or a dwarf, or a man with a defect in his sight or an itching disease or scab or crushed testicles; no man of the descendants of Aaron the priest who has a blemish, he shall not come near to offer the bread of his God, both of the most holy, and of the holy things.' "[11] In other words, the priest must be a whole, intact, perfect man.

"We have," concludes Douglas, "now laid a good basis for approaching the laws about clean and unclean meats. To be holy is to be whole, to be one; holiness is unity, integrity, perfection of the individual and of the kind. The dietary rules merely develop the metaphor of holiness on the same lines."[12]

The modern American drug laws have the same social function and same symbolic significance as had, for example, the dietary laws of the ancient Jews. The aim is still to be holy, which now means to be healthy; and to be healthy means to take those drugs prescribed by physicians (rabbis) and to avoid those prohibited by the state (God). As the dietary rules of the Jews developed the metaphor of holiness on the lines of prescribed and prohibited foods, so the drug rules of the Americans (and of other contemporary people) develop the metaphor of healthiness along the lines of prescribed and prohibited chemicals.

Such rules can, of course, be changed, without affecting their symbolic or ritual function. Indeed, such changes often express the changing needs of the community for a fresh ceremonial celebration of the ideas and images that sustain it. Thus the dietary laws of the Jews were changed by the Christians, as were their rules concerning the criteria of cleanliness required of the priest. Similarly, our drug laws were changed (in 1920 and 1933, those concerning alcohol; in 1937, those concerning marijuana), these changes serving only to enhance and revitalize their ritual function and significance.

The "answer," then, to our drug problem, insofar as one can meaningfully speak of such an answer, assuredly does not lie in bringing our drug laws in line with so-called scientific information.

It lies, instead, in demythologizing and de-ceremonializing our use and avoidance of drugs—something we are unlikely to accomplish without finding another, hopefully more humanly appropriate, vehicle for our symbolic coming together as a community of people.

4. COMMUNIONS, HOLY AND UNHOLY

The human need for social contact, for a communion with others of one's own kind, is second only to the organismic need for the satisfaction of the biological requirements for survival. In the satisfaction of this need for sociability, ceremony plays an indispensable part.

As the term "communion" implies, the celebration of the Lord's Supper through the Holy Communion at once symbolizes and realizes the joining together, in a community, of all those who participate in it. Indeed, the situation from which the ceremony originates, and which it memorializes, was itself a sociable communion of like-minded persons—namely, the Last Supper: "During supper, Jesus took bread, and having said the blessing he broke it and gave it to the disciples with the words: 'Take this and eat; this is my body.' Then he took a cup, and having offered thanks to God he gave it to them with the words: 'Drink from it, all of you. For this is my blood, the blood of the covenant, shed for many for the forgiveness of sins.' "[1]

To the non-Christian, the metaphorical or symbolic nature of this ritual is, of course, transparent: bread and wine *are not* the body and blood of Christ—they only *represent* them. Of course, we do not and cannot know what the phrases "this is my body . . . this is my blood" meant to Jesus or his disciples. They might have truly believed that the symbols *were* the referents—that bread and wine *were* body and blood. The point is that just as wine can, in the Holy Communion, *stand for* the blood of Christ—so alcohol can, in other contexts, in what some might regard as an Unholy Communion, *stand for* being powerful or being pauperized. And so it goes for other drugs, from marijuana to heroin. Men and women are capable of believing anything. This is simply a part, a consequence, of the human being's immense capacity to symbolize, to represent anything in the world by everything else. Once a person has made some sort of stable, symbolic connection between two things, that connection will influence his subsequent behavior and will generate its own "proof." This is why it is idle and foolish to try to "refute" religious, political, and similar beliefs with empirical arguments about referents that are symbols to the believer but not to the non-believer.

What is of special importance to us in this connection—that is, regarding our effort to distinguish between the ceremonial and chemical aspects of drugs—is that, in proportion as a person is a "believer," he believes that the symbol *is* the referent, or is at least prepared to conduct himself *as if* it were. Thus, to faithful Christians the Eucharist *is* the body and blood of Christ, or, in partaking of the Holy Communion, they act *as if* it were. To others, the Eucharist is simply a ceremonial prop; and these others—depending on the circumstances—may be considered non-believers, blaspheming Christians, infidels, heretics, and so forth.

In short, acceptance or non-acceptance of an identity between ceremonial symbol and ceremonial referent is a matter of membership in a community, and not a matter of fact or logic. This is not the place to examine whether and to what extent Christians throughout the ages believed in the literal identity, in the Eucharist, of bread and wine on the one hand and of the body and blood of Christ on the other; nor, indeed, would I be competent to undertake such an examination. It should suffice for us to note that one of the effects on Christianity of the Reformation was to weaken the literal interpretation of this ritual. As a result, the Council of Trent, in 1552, promulgated an authoritative interpretation—the first in the history of Christianity—of the ceremony of the Holy Communion. Called the "Doctrine of Transubstantiation," it is the Roman Catholic Church's official teaching on the subject of the conversion of the Bread and Wine into the Body and Blood of Christ in the Eucharist:

> If any one shall say that, in the Holy Sacrament of the Eucharist there remains, together with the Body and Blood of our Lord Jesus Christ, the substance of the Bread and Wine, and shall deny that wonderful and singular conversion of the whole substance of the Bread into (His) Body and of the Wine into (His) Blood, the species only of the Bread and Wine remaining—which conversion the Catholic Church most fittingly calls Transubstantiation—let him be anathema.[2]

What, then, have we here—again, from a non-Catholic point of view? A command, an insistence, to obliterate the difference between symbol and referent, between metaphorical and literal meaning. The Council decrees that the metaphor is the thing metaphorized—that bread is body and wine is blood. Why does it do so? I would think for two interrelated reasons. First, because parishioners and priests alike want to believe it is so, for only in this belief can they come together, in a "holy communion," not only with Jesus but with each other; because, in short, this belief is the ground on which their community as Christians rests. And second, because the Council understands that men have a limited capacity for seeing metaphor as metaphor, ritual as ritual; for, having seen it as such, they are likely to see it also as profane rather than sacred, as man-made rather than God-made, and hence lose faith in it and respect for the authority it symbolizes.

As in Christianity so also in our secular society; some shared beliefs are necessary to hold people together in groups. And many of our shared beliefs—and gatherings—have to do with drugs rather than with deities. Thus, just as in religions there are good and bad, benevolent and malevolent, deities—so in the secular religions of our drug age there are good and bad, therapeutic and toxic, drugs.

The adherents to our majority religions thus congregate at cocktail parties and "smokers"; and have elaborate ceremonies symbolizing the virtues of mixed drinks and wines, cigars and cigarettes, pipes and tobaccos, and so forth. These are the holy communions of our age.

Those who reject the doctrines of our principal religions and who cultivate instead various heretical faiths, congregate at pot and acid parties and at gatherings where heroin and other even more esoteric and forbidden drugs are used; and they too have elaborate ceremonies symbolizing the counter-virtues of marijuana and LSD, incense and Oriental mysticism, and so forth. These are the unholy communions of our age.

The ritual uses of alcohol—particularly of wine—are deeply embedded in the Judeo-Christian religions. The use of wine is first mentioned in the Bible in Genesis, where we learn that Noah planted a vineyard and became drunk on wine[3]—making him, one might suppose, history's first "alcoholic" or "drug abuser." The first unequivocally ceremonial use of wine cited in the Bible is also in Genesis. Melchizedek, king and high priest of Salem, uses it to offer a blessing on Abram: "Then Melchizedek, king of Salem, brought food and wine. He was priest of God Most High, and he pronounced this blessing on Abram."[4]

In Exodus, the specifications of the priestly ritual are set forth as follows: "In consecrating them to be my priests this is the rite to be observed . . . offer on the altar . . . a drink-offering of a quarter of a hin of wine for the first ram."[5] Similar prescriptions are given in Leviticus and in Numbers.[6]

And, skipping over numerous references in the Old and New Testaments, we come to the most significant biblical alcohol ceremonial of all, Jesus' use of wine in the Passover supper.[7] The first miracle by which Jesus reveals himself to his disciples concerns still another "miraculous transformation," this time of ceremonial water into ceremonial wine. Jesus is at a wedding at Cana-in-Galilee. The hosts have no wine. "There were six stone water-jars standing near, of the kind used for Jewish rites of purification; each held from twenty to thirty gallons. Jesus said to the servants 'Fill the jars with water,' and they filled them to the brim. 'Now draw some off,' he ordered, 'and take it to the steward of the feast'; and they did so. The steward tasted the water now turned into wine. . . . This deed at Cana-in-Galilee is the first of the signs by which Jesus revealed his glory and led his disciples to believe in him."[8]

It is clear that only in the first instance—where Noah uses wine alone and becomes intoxicated—is alcohol used for its purely pharmacological effect; in all of the other instances, it is used ceremonially—as part of a religious rite or as a celebration of a congregation of disciples, friends, and guests.

The ceremonial uses of marijuana are equally ancient. Herodotus describes people living on islands in the Araxes River who "meet together in companies," throw marijuana on the fire, then "sit around in a circle; and by inhaling the fruit that has been thrown on, they become intoxicated by the odor, just as the Greeks do by wine; and the more fruit is thrown on, the more intoxicated they become, until they rise up and dance, and betake themselves to singing."[9]

Snyder cites the following passages from "native literature" to illustrate the "religious role" of marijuana:

> To the Hindu the hemp plant is holy. A guardian lives in bhang. . . . Bhang is the joy giver, the sky flier, the heavenly guide, the poor man's heaven, the soother of grief. . . . No god or man is as good as the religious drinker of bhang. The students of the scriptures of Benares are given bhang before they sit to study. At Benares, Ujjaim and other holy places, yogis take deep draughts of bhang, that they may center their thoughts on the Eternal. . . . By the help of bhang ascetics pass days without food or drink. The supporting power of bhang has brought many a Hindu family safe through the miseries of famine.[10]

Most authorities state that the disapproval of marijuana use in the East originates with Christian missionaries. Thus, J. Campbell Oman notes that Christian missionaries often describe Hindu saints as living "in a state of perpetual intoxication and call this stupefaction, which arises from smoking intoxicating herbs, fixing the mind on god."[11] The Brahmins of India are habitual users of marijuana (bhang), and view their god Shiva as a bhang drinker.

In the light of this sort of historical and cultural evidence, Snyder cites this warning—issued by a "native writer" whose views were cited by the Indian Hemp Drug Commission Report of 1893 —concerning efforts to prohibit the use of bhang in India:

> To forbid or even seriously to restrict the use of so holy and gracious a herb as the hemp would cause widespread suffering and annoyance and to large bands of worshipped ascetics deep seeded anger. It would rob the people of solace in discomfort, of cure in sickness, of a guardian whose gracious protection saves them from the attacks of evil influences . . . so grand a result, so tiny a sin![12]

One of the most important aspects of ceremonial drug use is that the desire for the drug is experienced as issuing from the very depth of the user; whereas, in the case of the therapeutic use of drugs, the user experiences external necessity, or even compul-

sion, as the motive for drug taking. It is precisely this experience
of an inner need or "craving" that justifies our placing this behavior in the same class with other patterns of religious conduct
and observance: what all these behaviors—that is, drug use recognized as religious, drug "addiction," and habitual "drug abuse"—
share with other kinds of religious behaviors is the experience of
a profound inner desire or urge, whose satisfaction gratifies the
user's deepest sense of existence or being in the world. And herein,
too, lies the reason why both the religious fanatic and the "dope
fiend" go to such great lengths to satisfy their desires; and why
each feels fully justified in the moral righteousness of his conduct.
This "call" or "craving"—which to the observer seems to come
from without, from the voice of God or the lure of a drug, but
which to the subject comes from within, from the recognition of
the subject's "calling" or from the conviction that only with the
drug is he "whole"—must, moreover, be contrasted, if we are to
appreciate its real import, with the universal human experience it
opposes, and indeed tries to annihilate; namely, the experience of
helplessness and powerlessness and of being manipulated by external agents and their hostile interests.[13]

In the countless ceremonial uses of drugs and in the oppositions
to them, a fundamental polarity and "problem" inherent in human
nature is dramatized and ritualized: namely, the struggle between
man controlling himself and man controlled by alien powers, between self-reliance and reliance on others, between autonomy and
heteronomy.[14]

How deeply, and how ceremonially, alcohol and tobacco are
entrenched into the lives of English-speaking people is revealed in
the following lines, quoted from Keith Thomas' fine historical
study of "popular beliefs in sixteenth and seventeenth century
England": Drink "was built into the fabric of social life. It played
a part in nearly every public and private ceremony, every commercial bargain, every craft ritual, every private occasion of
mourning or rejoicing. . . . As a Frenchman observed in 1672,
there was no business which could be done in England without
pots of beer."[15] Thomas estimates that at the end of the seven-

teenth century the per capita consumption of beer in England was "higher than anything known in modern times."[16]

In part, of course, alcohol was used as "an essential narcotic which anaesthetised men against the strains of contemporary life." It flowed freely at times of the plague: bearers carrying the corpses to their graves were often drunk. And at executions, Thomas writes, "drink was always offered to the condemned: the witch Anne Bodenham, who was executed at Salisbury in 1653, kept asking for drink and would have died drunk if her persecutors had allowed her."[17] As a fifteenth-century heretic revealingly remarked: "There was more good in a cask of ale than in the four gospels."[18]

Thomas' observations on tobacco are equally interesting and relevant. "Smoking was introduced to England early in the reign of Elizabeth I and had become well-established by the time of her death. At first there was an attempt to represent tobacco as being taken for medicinal purposes, but the pretence soon became unconvincing."[19] The tobacco habit spread rapidly, per capita consumption rising from less than an ounce at the beginning of the seventeenth century to nearly two pounds at the end of it.[20] Although it is not his main concern, Thomas is well aware of the ceremonial functions of smoking. He notes that "tobacco must have done something to steady the nerves of Stuart Englishmen," and adds that it may have helped to foster the characteristic British talent for political compromise. Finally, he cites Christopher Marlowe's telling remark that "Holy Communion would have been much better being administered in a tobacco pipe."[21]

Surely it is difficult to evade the conclusion that the use of alcohol and the use of tobacco have become deeply ingrained habits in Christian and English-speaking countries, and that we therefore consider these substances good; and that, because the use of marijuana (hashish) and the use of opium are pagan and foreign habits, we consider these substances bad.

The view that alcohol, tobacco, and coffee are the secular sacraments of our chemical ceremonies is readily supported by observations anyone can make. A few dramatic illustrations of it should suffice here.

In a *Playboy* interview, Tennessee Williams remarked that ". . . for a long time, I couldn't walk down a street unless I could see a bar—not because I wanted a drink but because I wanted the security of knowing it was there."[22] The replacement of the church by the bar, of the priest by the bartender, of the holy water by the alcohol, and of the communion with God by the communion with fellow patrons is here rendered with unmistakable clarity. Alcohol and the social paraphernalia associated with drinking have thus served a truly religious function for Mr. Williams, as the following passage from the same interview also shows: "I've never wanted a Cadillac. In fact, I don't want any car at all. I used to get panicky on the California freeway. I always carried a little flask with me and, if I forgot it, I would go into a panic."[23] The flask of alcohol evidently had the same function for Mr. Williams as a religious icon would have for a formally religious person.

As there are pure or holy objects in magic and religion, there must also be polluted or unholy ones. Here is how this dichotomy is seen and articulated as part of our contemporary "common sense." "Alcohol is a good that can be abused," writes a reader in the letters column of *National Review*. "With dope it is otherwise. . . . Taking dope is a form of mutilation, and mutilation is forbidden by natural law."[24]

Let me now support my suggestion that we oppose illicit drugs not because they are the wrong chemicals but because they are the wrong ceremonials, by citing a quite ordinary newspaper account of our efforts to control the "heroin epidemic." If read with an eye on the possible parallels between drugs and religions, between ritual drug use and ritual religious observance, it will be apparent that what we *call* a "war against drug abuse" is actually a war to eliminate, everywhere if possible, the use of drugs of which we disapprove, and at the same time to encourage everywhere the use of drugs of which we approve.

In a story in *The New York Times* on the latest opium war in Asia—this time, of course, to prohibit rather than to promote the drug—we learn how the peasants in Laos resist attempts to curtail their traditional habit of cultivating poppy and using opium as a folk medicine. Reporting from Nam Keung in Laos, the correspondent for the *Times* writes that "under intense pressure from the United States Embassy, including the threat to cut off American aid, the Laotian Government last year reversed its traditional policy and banned the production, sale, and consumption of opium, known in Laos as 'flower medicine.' "[25]

To the Laotians, this is, of course, an infringement of their liberties, and a very serious one at that. " 'It is hard for my people to understand why they should stop growing opium because they are told that it kills Americans thousands of miles away in a strange country,' Chao La, the Yao chief of Nam Keung, told a delegation of Laotian Cabinet ministers, legislators, and American officials who visited his village earlier this week."[26]

The interference by American officials in the daily lives of the Laotians is then set forth; and we learn that, in the name of an "anti-narcotic program . . . backed by $2.9 million in United States aid," the following measures have been taken:

1. Sixteen American "customs and narcotics experts" now operate in Laos; fifteen local drug traders have been arrested.

2. "About 1,500 of the estimated 20,000 drug addicts in Laos have been treated at a Buddhist temple in Thailand, and at a newly opened detoxification clinic that uses methadone in Vientiane."

3. "The Agency for International Development is helping build new roads into opium growing areas"—ostensibly "to improve the access of alternative crops to markets," but perhaps more likely to improve the surveillance capabilities of the narcotics agents.

This arrogant destruction of "alien" customs and ceremonies is, as crusades always are, carried out pitilessly, and only for the good of the victims themselves. "To the Yao residents of Nam Keung, a small settlement of bamboo and thatch houses perched on a bluff over the Mekong River, the controversy over opium seems incomprehensible and unfair. For them as for many of Laos' manifold ethnic groups, opium has long been the best remedy for all ills, from diarrhea to menstrual cramps and tuberculosis. 'We are a poor people who do not have easy lives,' Chao La, the village chief, told the visiting delegation of Laotian and American officials. The visitors—who included Edgar Buell, 'Mister Pop,' the nearly legendary A.I.D. officer who has worked with the mountain tribes of Laos since 1959—hoped to persuade the Yao to give up growing opium."[27]

If "Mr. Pop" cannot persuade the Yao to do what, save for American coercion, they have no conceivable reason for doing, then he, or his employers, will perhaps make them an offer they won't be able to refuse. I cite this story—which to me epitomizes the moral degeneracy of our war against narcotics—partly because it presents a vivid picture of this war, and partly because it reveals so starkly that this war is not just a struggle *against* "their drugs" but also a struggle *for* "ours."

Before returning to their home base, the Laotian Cabinet ministers, legislators, and American officials—including, presumably, "Mr. Pop" himself—gave the native Asiatic drug abusers a demonstration of the proper Western drug ceremonial: "After downing dozens of glasses of deadly home-brewed corn whisky known as lao-lao, the delegation left Nam Keumg without being quite certain what had been agreed to."[28]

I think what had been agreed to is entailed quite clearly in what this whole "visit," as a social ceremony, symbolizes. The powerful foreign invader appears in the village and offers tempting bribes for the destruction of traditional customs. (We might substitute Buddhism or Christianity for opium to get this picture into proper focus.) Implicit in the visit, and in the powers and propensities of the visitors, is the further message that if the bribes are rejected, more direct and painful means may be used to exact compliance. Finally, the invader leaves, but not before celebrating his own drug ceremonial, thus making it clear that his real aim is to convert the natives from their drug (opium) to his (alcohol).

Here, then, in microcosm—in a tiny Laotian village—we see the American anti-narcotic crusade writ large. Like Christians burning mosques and temples to spread the word of Jesus, modern drug-abuseologists burn crops to spread the use of alcohol.

Furthermore, in contrast to the war in Vietnam, which has been condemned by countless Americans and by even more non-Americans, this war in Asia (and elsewhere) has received nothing but praise and support. I am not aware of any political party or group anywhere in the world having denounced, on principle, this brutal—and both morally and medically quite unjustifiable—invasion of other people's rights to grow poppy and use opium. In my opinion, this pseudomedical crusade—supported alike by capitalist and Communist countries—may, in the long run, prove to be more damaging to the cause of human freedom and dignity than have any of the armed conflicts of our age.

What exists today is nothing less than a worldwide quasi-medical pogrom against opium and the users of opiates. The reason why this persecution is worldwide is simple: the "conversion" from opium to alcohol symbolizes the transformation of a people from a shameful past of "backwardness" to a shining present and future of "modernity," and is supported by all three of the world's superpowers—the U.S., the U.S.S.R., and China. (The Chinese have, as far as I know, taken only the first step in this process: they have banned the use of opium; they have not yet taken the second step, that is, they have not yet adopted alcohol as the proper recreational drug and rich source of governmental revenue.)

Until the 1950s, opium use was legal in Iran. In the following account by Henry Kamm of the way opium was used, the similarities with alcohol use are dramatic, even though Kamm is, of course, not trying to make the point I am. "Many of the homes of the Teheran upper class used to have a well-appointed room to which male guests retired after dinner and from which the sweet smell of first-rate smoking opium soon wafted out to the ladies in the drawing room. Those who liked opium entered the room for a sociable pipe or two; those who didn't stayed with the ladies, very much like some take an after-dinner brandy when the tray is brought around and others pass it up. No stigma was attached."[29]

The last comment seems gratuitous and may even be misleading. From all that I know and have read about such matters, it would seem more likely that the stigma was the other way around: it was probably attached to those who were not "men enough" to smoke opium. This supposition is confirmed by the fact that, as Kamm tells it, ". . . most teahouses used to sell opium, and even the Iranian Parliament had a lounge that, while not an opium den, served as a place where deputies gathered to smoke opium."[30]

The general who led the war against this shameful Iranian habit is himself an Iranian—a physician, to be sure, and of course American-trained. He is Dr. Jehanshaw Saleh, who, as Health Minister, prevailed on the Shah to prohibit the cultivation and use of opium in 1955. To do this, he had to relabel all opium users as "addicts," a coup he was evidently able to pull off. "Before [the ban]," Kamm quotes Dr. Saleh as saying, "if you looked at Parliament, you saw opium addicts."[31] Unmistakably, one way to succeed in the world of politics and social science is to malign, in just the right way, your own country, its people, and its leaders: one must not malign them (even if it is true) by saying that they are unpatriotic, stupid, or steal the taxpayers' money; instead, one must malign them by saying that they are "sick"—opium addicts, alcohol addicts, mentally ill—and then one will be hailed as a savior of the country whose most important traditions and values one has helped to destroy with a mere "diagnosis."

Did the prohibition of opium in Iran succeed? Not exactly. It created an immediate and immense illicit market in opium, and other troubles as well. But none of this impaired Dr. Saleh's or the Shah's greatness in the least. They have since basked in the glory of the following consequences of the 1955 ban: in 1969, they reintroduced the use of opium into Iran under medical supervision; they "reintroduced limited cultivation of the poppy under strict supervision"; they "recognized" opium use as an "addiction" and "provided for an expanded treatment program—and for the threat of the firing squad for trafficking and illegal use."[32] If this scenario sounds familiar, the fault is not mine but history's.

Iran has maintained itself as a nation for more than two thousand years, with its people using opium in moderation, mainly to help them endure their harsh and barren lives. Why, then, did it have to enact Opium Prohibition all of a sudden in 1955? "Prohibition was motivated," writes Kamm, "largely by prestige reasons. At a time of modernization, which in most developing countries means imitation of Western models, the use of opium was considered a shameful hangover of a dark Oriental past. It did not fit with the image of an awakening, Westernizing Iran that the Shah was creating."[33]

The "imitation of Western models" is the key phrase here. This imitation includes the following main elements: the substitution of alcohol for opium; the medicalization of certain personal habits and cultural traditions, especially those which the state wants to prohibit; and the introduction of medical methods of social control. Though somewhat late, Iran has found its own Guillotins and Rushes. Observes Kamm: "Dr. Saleh [a Syracuse-educated gynecologist who is a senator] and Dr. Azarakhsh [Director General of the Iranian Ministry of Health] deplore the smoking of opium because as physicians as well as patriots it pains them to see Persians on a large scale indulge in a habit that is unhealthy. 'It's like you bring up a child until he's 14 years old and then you cut his head off,' Dr. Saleh said."[34]

Of course, Dr. Saleh is still a little amateurish in the way he dramatizes the consequences of the opium habit. But, after all, he is a gynecologist, not a psychiatrist. Although he claims that using opium is an "addiction," he really prefers shooting people who mess around with such things to treating them. Dr. Saleh and Dr. Azarakhsh are, says Kamm, "unhappy that the resumption of opium-growing after 14 years of total ban and the official sanction of registered addiction seemingly restore some respectability to a habit they hate."[35] But Kamm does not say, and there is no reason to believe, that these "patriotic" doctors are unhappy that in the last three years alone, 160 "pushers" have been summarily shot.

The evidence strongly suggests that where Jesus on the Cross may have failed to convert "others" to "our" ways, alcohol in the bottle may yet succeed. Remarking on "Teheran's swingers"—on those, that is, who have adapted most successfully to the Iranian opium prohibition—Kamm writes: "Illustrating the modernity of his class, the young man took a sip from his whisky and soda forbidden by the Koran."[36] "Modernity" here really means "drinking alcohol"—like the Americans and the Russians drink it; like the English, the French, the Italians, and the Hungarians drink it; and like all the other "normal" people of the world drink it.

Perhaps when everyone will speak English (or Russian), use the metric system, diet, sedate himself with whisky or vodka, stimulate himself with cigarettes and erotic advertising, and will be medicated by his state-employed doctor with state-approved anorexics, anti-depressants, ataractics, and yet-to-be-discovered anti-thinking agents—perhaps then everything will be all right. Obviously, we have put our faith in the wrong Savior. Now our "friends" and "imitators" are showing us that the true Savior is not Christ but Chemistry.

As living organisms, we perceive and refract physical reality through our sense organs; and as human beings, we perceive and refract social reality through those parts of our bodies that make us specifically human—namely, our organs of speech, hearing, and the higher centers of the brain that subserve the symbolic functions of language. It is not surprising, then, that where the symbolic function of human conduct plays an important role—as in religion, art, and politics—the role of language in that type of conduct, and in its interpretation, will be equally important.

Culturally accepted drugs have traditionally been promoted, and today continue to be promoted, as the symbols of adulthood and maturity. Tobacco and alcohol—and, indeed, even coffee and tea—are substances that are permitted to adults but, as a rule, not to children. This makes these drugs, ipso facto, symbols of maturity and competence. Formerly, men sported large cigars clenched between their teeth—much as they sported large pocket watches on gold chains in their vest pockets—as the symbols of their adult masculinity. The large masculine cigars have now been largely replaced by smaller bisexual ones—rolled hunks of tobacco advertised equally for both men and "emancipated" women, symbolizing the adulthood of each in contrast to the infantilism of children for whom the sale of such cigars remains prohibited. Among tobacco products, cigarettes, of course, continue to remain the leading symbols of maturity and sophistication, a role they share about evenly with beer and liquor—nicotine and alcohol constituting the two major socially approved and promoted drugs throughout the "civilized" world.

The social approval of certain recreational drugs is reflected and sustained by the language we use to describe the various activities associated with their manufacture, sale, and use. People who make liquor are businessmen, not the "members of an international ring of alcohol refiners"; people who sell liquor are retail merchants, not "pushers"; and people who buy liquor are citizens, not "dope fiends." The same things go for tobacco, coffee, and tea.

The use of medicinal, rather than recreational, drugs is promoted quite differently, but the same principles apply. Aspirin, tranquilizers, drugs to make a person sleepy or alert—all these are promoted under the banner of medical science. People are told that whatever "ails" them—and it does not matter in the least what it is, from boredom with one's job to conflict with one's mother-in-law, or all the countless metaphorical diseases called "mental illness"—is a *disease* for which the proper remedy is this or that specific drug. All this is, of course, a colossal fraud. But, then, it is no greater fraud than telling people that whatever ails them is a sin for which the proper remedy is prayer—and perhaps some sacrifice to God or payment to the Church. Indeed, the clinical panacea is often a faithful replica of the clerical one.

Just as culturally approved drugs have generally been promoted as symbols of maturity, and their habitual use as proof of competence in life's games—so culturally disapproved drugs have generally been prohibited as the symbols of immaturity, and their habitual use as proof of incompetence in life's games and hence the symptom of mental disease or moral debauchment or both. Thus, in the literature of official psychiatry, the dogma that drug addiction is a mental illness is never questioned; nor is the belief that a person becomes an addict because of an "underlying defect" in his personality. In short, the psychiatric mythology concerning drug abuse is an exact replica of the psychiatric mythology concerning self-abuse (masturbation).[37]

This sort of psychiatric interpretation is, of course, circular. Traditional psychiatry has accepted the conventional definition of a certain kind of behavior—masturbation, the use of illegal drugs, and so forth—as a type of disease falling specifically within the province of the "psychiatric physician." Having done so, all that remained for psychiatry was to establish its "etiology": a defect in the depth of the psyche; describe the course of the "untreated disease": steady deterioration leading straight to the insane asylum;

and prescribe its "treatment": psychiatric coercion with or without the use of additional, "therapeutic" drugs (heroin for morphine; methadone for heroin; antabuse for alcohol).

Thus, a critique of the languages of drug use and drug avoidance cannot proceed very far before one is compelled to observe that there is, in fact, no such thing as "drug addiction." To be sure, some people do take drugs that the authorities do not want them to take; and some people do become used to taking certain substances, or become habituated to them; and the various substances which people take may be legal or illegal, relatively harmless or quite harmful. But the difference between someone "using a drug" and his being "addicted" to it is not a matter of fact, but a matter of our moral attitude and political strategy toward him. Indeed, we might, and must, go further than this, and note that the very identification of a substance as a drug or not a drug is not a matter of fact but a matter of moral attitude and political strategy: tobacco, in common parlance, is not considered to be a drug, but marijuana is; gin is not, but Valium is. Here, now, briefly is how those who wish to wage war on drugcraft use the language of loathing to enlist recruits for their cause.

The title of a newspaper column by Art Linkletter, the famous entertainer, asks: "How do I tell if my child is hooked?"[38] The title of a magazine article by Ira Mothner, senior editor of *Look*, asks: "How can you tell if your child is taking drugs?"[39] The language of these pieces, beginning with their titles and ending with their exhortation to deceive and coerce in the best of all possible causes, narcotizes our moral sensibility: authors and readers lull each other into a tacit acceptance—never questioned and indeed quite unquestionable—that, in the holy medical crusade against addiction, trying to control other people by any means is not only morally proper but indeed praiseworthy. It is thus first taken for granted, and then reinforced, that parents ought to spy on their children; that doctors should play detective vis-à-vis their patients; and that the American government should self-righteously interfere in the domestic affairs of all other countries—if such interventions are "necessary" to "save" people from the "plague of heroin addiction."

In our day, nowhere is the language of scapegoating more clearly displayed than in the way we write and talk about drug use and drug avoidance. The proximal scapegoat is the "dangerous drug"; a slightly more distal one is "the addict" who "infects" others with his "disease"; and the ultimate one is "the pusher." This addiction-mongering rhetoric has now been escalated to an invocation of a "doomsday" of "infection," and to the demand that all other human interests and values be subordinated to a fanatical quest for freedom from the poppy. Many of the foremost political, scientific, and literary figures throughout the world have joined this frenzied chorus.

A headline in the *Saturday Review* asks: "Ten years to doomsday?"[40] In the article we learn that French Interior Minister Raymond Marcellin believes that "the vast majority of French people, young and old, are allergic to drugs."[41] In the same article, Dr. Gunnar Myrdal, famed Swedish political economist, declares that international agreements "on drug control are an absolute necessity."[42] Presumably he does not intend to classify nicotine or alcohol as "drugs." Not to be outdone, the highest-ranking American expert quoted in this article states flatly: "Nothing is more important than drugs."[43] This remarkable view is expressed by Mr. Myles Ambrose, who, when this article was published, was head of the United States Bureau of Customs, and perhaps on the strength of his convictions, was soon promoted to be Special Consultant to the President for Drug Abuse Law Enforcement.

Not quite two years later, Mr. Ambrose provided a public expression of his devotion to his job. This was in the form of a Letter to the Editor in *The New York Times*, written jointly with Dr. Jerome H. Jaffe, Special Consultant to the President for Narcotics and Dangerous Drugs. Their letter was written about a year after the American anti-drug warriors succeeded in pressuring the Turkish government to ban the cultivation of the poppy, a success that only galvanized the prohibitionists into still greater exertions of their will to power. "Few of us," write Dr. Jaffe and Mr. Ambrose, "had 'illusions' that the agreement with Turkey to end production of opium would 'solve' the problem. . . . It is necessary to understand that a very small portion—perhaps 5 percent—of the world's opium production is required to supply our heroin addict population. The major thrust of the Federal effort is to develop effective prevention programs and to see that treatment is available to all who want it. . . . . President Nixon has requested $729 million for the war on drug abuse in fiscal 1972, a 1,000 percent increase over the Government's expenditure of $65 million in 1969."[44]

Obviously, addiction has been the ·glamor stock of the late sixties and early seventies, and addiction mongering the only true growth industry in America during these years. The profitable nature of the war on addiction has, of course, been noted by numerous observers, most of whom, however, do not question the assumption that drug addiction is a disease, and therefore accept the proposition that it can be "treated." Marion Sanders' comments are typical of this sort of sobriety that stops short of thinking the unthinkable—namely, that the whole business of addiction mongering is a gigantic hoax, a socially and professionally validated racket. She writes: "Nineteen-seventy may well be remembered as the year of the great drug panic, the year when addiction was a permanent theme in the press and on TV and when government officials and office seekers made instant headlines by leading a 'massive attack' on the problem . . . the treatment of addicts has become a growth industry with proponents of various theories fiercely vying for public funds to support their enterprises. Most 'private' addiction treatment programs in New York are heavily dependent on government support."[45]

In the English-speaking world today, the principal places where people commune or congregate to articulate, affirm, and experience a feeling of conviviality, of belonging to a group of like-minded persons—where each person's habit validates that of every other—are the bar, pub, or tavern. In America and in England, there are far more places for drinking than for worshipping; many more bartenders than clergymen or physicians. In Milwaukee, Wisconsin, for example, there were 13,100 bartenders in 1972, or one bartender for every 55 persons in the city.[46] Can anyone doubt that the ceremonial celebration of communality—of wholeness, goodness, togetherness—is now articulated through pretzels and beer, rather than through bread and wine?

Criticism of anti-drug laws and so-called narcotics controls is often misinterpreted as approval or endorsement of drug use or drug addiction. Those who so interpret my position—or any position of laissez faire and tolerance with respect to drug use—do so because they implicitly subscribe to the principle that anyone who does not support their position supports their adversary's. Nothing could be farther from the truth. I regard tolerance with respect to drugs as wholly analogous to tolerance with respect to religion. To be sure, a Christian advocating religious tolerance at the height of the Inquisition would himself have been accused of heresy. Today, however, no one would misinterpret his position as an endorsement or advocacy of a non-Christian religion or of atheism. The fact that a contemporary American's, and especially physician's, advocacy of tolerance with respect to drugs is generally viewed as an endorsement or support of undisciplined licentiousness in the use of "dangerous drugs" signifies that we are now at the height of an "anti-narcotic" inquisition.

II. Pharmacomythology: Medicine as Magic

5. LICIT AND ILLICIT HEALING: PERSECUTIONS FOR WITCHCRAFT AND DRUGCRAFT

In every society, people look to certain authorities for curing disease. As soon as a society reaches a sufficient degree of complexity, these authorities will tend to monopolize the healing function: they will then define themselves, and will be defined by the holders of power, as the only accredited or licit healers, all others being cast in the category of unaccredited or illicit healers or quacks.

It will be instructive to consider some of the similarities between the medieval wars against witchcraft and the modern wars against drugcraft. In each of these contests we witness a ritualized dramatization of the defiance and defense of the dominant social ethic; a concealed conflict between indigenous or illicit healers and their accredited or professionalized competitors; and, ultimately, a struggle between individuals aspiring to care for themselves by contracting for their own healing, and collectivities or states insisting upon caring for their members by subjecting them to procedures they define as therapeutic. Our contemporary drug problems thus cannot be understood without paying proper attention to the subtle but powerful tensions between accredited and unaccredited healers, physicians and quacks, licit and illicit drugs, scientific medicine and folk medicine—tensions that have profound emotional as well as economic ramifications.

Traditional accounts of the history of medicine trace its origins from Hippocrates and Galen in the ancient world; through the labors of "regular" physicians—mainly Arabs and Jews—in the Dark Ages; and thence to the birth of "scientific" medicine during the Renaissance and Enlightenment. Through a significant omission, this account falsifies the history of medicine: it ignores the role of the medieval "white witch." (The "white witches" were women trusted for their supposed powers to help and heal, as opposed to the "black witches," who were feared for their supposed powers to cause misfortune, illness, and death.) It is revealing, indeed, that just as in the Jewish history of creation, mankind has a divine father but no mother at all; and as in the Christian history of it, mankind has a divine father but only a human mother; so in the male-medical history of medicine, this discipline too has lofty fathers but no mothers. In this case, we can confidently assert that this male parthenogenetic fantasy of the birth of medicine is just that—a fantasy. The fact is that, although the noble priest-physicians of antiquity are no doubt the far-distant ancestors of the modern medical scientist, his next of kin is his mother—the medieval white witch.[1]

To understand the role of the white witch—often called the "wisewoman"—as a healer, we must remember that in the Middle Ages medicine, like other branches of learning, was in a state of arrest. As Jules Michelet puts it: "With the exception of Arab or Jewish physicians, hired at great cost by the rich, medical treatment was unknown—the people could only crowd to the church doors for aspersion with holy water."[2]

The licit healers were thus the priests, and the correct, socially accredited methods of healing consisted of prayer, fasting, and the appropriate applications of holy water. Naturally, this did not satisfy many people, not only because they knew that the rich used physicians inaccessible to the poor, but also because they knew that there were herbs and potions, incantations and other magic rituals, offered by the "unlicensed" or "indigenous" therapists of their day, the witches. As Pennethorne Hughes points out, "Jews were branded as usurers because no one but a Jew was permitted to lend money under the medieval system, and they were allowed few other professions. In the same way, witches had largely a monopoly of the powers of healing—the dual powers of healing and harming—because of the medieval injunction against medicine."[3] The monopoly Hughes refers to was, of course, an illicit one, like that now enjoyed in America by the Mafia (or "organized crime") with respect to the importation and distribution of heroin. This, of course, is only one of many similarities, as we shall presently see, between witchcraft and drugcraft, and between the wars against them.

The witches themselves both used pharmacologically active substances (which I shall henceforth call "drugs") and gave them to others—another similarity between them and the contemporary users of illicit drugs. The legendary witches' brews condensed all of the complex and even antithetical uses to which the pharmacological technology of witchcraft could be put: the brew would bestow magical powers on the witch who took it, and could be used to poison the healthy or cure the sick. Moreover, there is solid evidence to support the view that, although the witch's curative powers rested in part on magic (that is, on her "patients'" belief in her ability to heal), these women also possessed numerous pharmacologically active substances and knew how to use them. For example, in 1527, Paracelsus, considered one of the greatest physicians of his time, declared publicly that "he had learned from the Sorceresses [white witches] all he knew."[4]

In Margaret Murray's classic *The Witch-Cult in Western Europe,* A. J. Clark gives specific information about the composition of an ointment that witches used in connection with their celebration of the "sabbat." The psychoactive—or, as we might now call them, the "psychedelic"—effects of these ointments are obvious, and remarkably similar to those now often attributed to LSD.

The use of ointments, rubbed into the skin, is, of course, a part of many religions. This practice was thus partly ceremonial and partly chemical in nature, inasmuch as certain substances were absorbed into the body through the unbroken, or more often broken, skin. Concerning the "flying ointment" used by European witches, Clark has this to say:

> The three formulae for "flying" ointment used by witches are as follows: 1. Parsley, water of aconite, poplar leaves, and soot. 2. Water parsnip, sweet flag, cinquefoil, bat's blood, deadly nightshade, and oil. 3. Baby's fat, juice of water parsnip, aconite, cinquefoil, deadly nightshade, and soot.
> These prescriptions show that the society of witches had a very creditable knowledge of the art of poisoning; aconite and deadly nightshade or belladonna are two of the three most poisonous plants growing freely in Europe; the third is hemlock, and in all probability "persil" refers to hemlock and not the harmless parsley, which it resembles closely.[5]

In what follows, Clark tells us something not only about the pharmacological competence of the witches, but also about the historical antecedents of the contemporary problem of drug abuse and drug controls:

> Aconite was one of the best known poisons in ancient times; indeed, it was so extensively used by professional poisoners in Rome during the Empire that a law was passed making its cultivation a capital offense. . . . The use of belladonna as a poison was also known in classical times; fourteen of the berries have been known to produce death; a moderate dose will produce wild excitement and delirium. Hemlock is also a well-known ancient poison. . . . There is no doubt, therefore, about the efficacy of these prescriptions and their ability to produce physiological effects. . . . I cannot say whether any of these drugs would produce the impression of flying, but I consider the use of aconite interesting in this respect. Irregular action of the heart in a person falling asleep produces the well-known sensation of suddenly falling through space, and it seems quite possible that the combination of a delirifacient like belladonna with a drug producing irregular action of the heart like aconite might produce the sensation of flying.[6]

In short, we have, in this account of drug use by medieval witches, the precursors of the illusion of flying, or of being able to fly, now attributed to LSD; and also of witches in social roles comparable not only to today's indigenous healers but also to those of illicit drug users ("addicts") and sellers ("pushers"). It would appear, moreover, that the impressions of flying—and indeed of false or distorted impressions of one's own body or surroundings—are not so much drug-specific as they are situation-specific: they occur with the use of all sorts of drugs where a feeling of exaltation is the result the initiate is expected to experience. Thus, Hughes remarks that "Persian dervishes and others have obtained the same sort of effect [as the witches had] from hashish, passing from exaltation to complete hallucination. Under the influence of this drug, a little stone is said to appear as a huge block, a gutter as a wide stream, a path as a wide endless road. The addict fancies he has wings, and that he can rise from the ground."[7]

Before concluding these brief remarks on white witches, to whom modern medicine owes so much and yet whose worth it tries to deny and whose very existence it wants to ignore—I want to call attention to modern medicine's startlingly similar attitude toward the poppy, to which, too, it owes so much and yet whose worth it now tries to deny and whose very existence it now wants to annihilate.

For millennia, opium has served as mankind's, and as medicine's, best—most effective and safest—pain killer and mood elevator. But opium, like the indigenous healer, is simple and unpretentious: the dried juice of the poppy. No chemist, no pharmaceutical industry, no physician is needed to produce it or to administer it. This, I submit, is one of the important reasons why modern medicine has so ungratefully turned its back on the poppy, just as it had, earlier, on the wisewoman: each reminds the arrogant "doctor"—aspiring to control rather than to cure his patient—of his lowly origins; and worse, each threatens him with displacement by the indigenous healer, by folk medicine, and by the efforts of the sick person to cure himself through self-medication—all this making the physician dispensable and insecure. This, then, is also one of the important reasons why the modern physician has embraced synthetic pain killers and mood changers: there can be no Darvon or Valium without chemists, pharmaceutical industries, and physicians to prescribe them! This makes the modern physician appear as a scientist, not a magician; and it makes him indispensable—as the protector of the patient from the quack, and even from himself!

It is against this background that we should view, and that I wish to examine, the parallels between licit and illicit drugs, licit and illicit healers, and the contest between them.

Those who practiced witchcraft engaged in taking and giving drugs, and so do those who now practice drugcraft—that is, those who take and give illicit drugs. In both cases, the deviants are persecuted and punished not only for what they *do* but also for who they *are:* defiant members of a "counter-culture."

It is unnecessary here to repeat the facts of the famous witch hunts. It seems clear, however—both from the evidence of history and from that of human nature—that the war against the witches was waged so ferociously partly because the witches threatened the oligarchic powers of the priests, in the same way that the war against pushers is waged so ferociously partly because the pushers threaten the oligarchic powers of the physicians. It is a remarkable, and relevant, fact that the first person to be executed in the colony of Massachusetts Bay was Margaret Jones, a "female physician" accused of witchcraft.[8]

Formerly, in theocratic societies, only the priest was allowed to practice healing. If the witch practiced healing, she was condemned regardless of the consequences of her efforts: if she harmed her client, she was punished for being an evildoer; if she helped him, she was punished for seducing the faithful and bewitching the innocent. Today, in therapeutic societies, only the physician is allowed to dispense "dangerous drugs." If anyone else does so, he is called a "pusher," and is again condemned and punished regardless of the consequences of his efforts.

The result of the medieval rivalry between witches and priests was the Inquisition, with all its complex and far-reaching consequences—in particular, the development of a powerful group of witch mongers, whose vested interest it became to produce ever more witches in order to make themselves ever more indispensable and wealthy. The modern persecution of drug abusers and pushers has generated a similar Medical Inquisition, with complex and far-reaching consequences—among them, the development of a powerful group of addiction mongers whose vested interest is to produce ever more drug abusers in order to make themselves ever more indispensable and wealthy.

Such developments are, indeed, inevitable—because they are built into the "fabric" of society; and because one of the obvious characteristics of that fabric is that important and identifiable social activities are, and have always been, institutionalized. Religion is institutionalized as a priesthood; medicine, as a profession of physicians; the dispensing of drugs, as pharmacy. Similarly, the war on heretics and witches was institutionalized as the Inquisition. And the war on dangerous drugs, addicts, and pushers—that is, on drugcraft—is institutionalized as the Bureau of Narcotics and Dangerous Drugs, the National Institute of Mental Health, and other agencies and groups, teaming up for a war against drugcraft.

Like the Inquisition, the Medical Holy War on drug abuse is international in scope. And as the Inquisition had two principal centers, one in Rome and the other in Spain, the Medical Inquisition also has two principal centers, one in Washington and the other in Switzerland. The true spiritual center of this holy war may be said to be in the American capital, and particularly in its suburban National Institutes of This and That Disease and Drug. Out of these centers, too, come the master plans for the production and distribution of the Medical Holy Water—Methadone—to counteract the Heretical Witch's Brew of Heroin.

The center for the international operations of the Medical Inquisition is located in Switzerland, mainly in Geneva, in the offices of the various anti-addiction and anti-drug abuse bureaucracies of the United Nations. Needless to say, these agencies are not concerned with drug habits such as drinking, smoking, or "methadone maintenance," but are concerned only with those habits that are induced and maintained by people unsupervised by doctors and involving substances which the United Nations classifies as "illicit drugs."

The Church, Michelet remarks, "declares, in the fourteenth century, that if a woman dare cure *without having studied, she is a witch and must die.*"[9] Of course, "studying" here refers to studying the Scriptures and qualifying, in effect, as a priest. In the same way, in the twentieth century, Medicine declares that if a man, woman, or child dares to dispense drugs without having a medical license—and dispenses a "dangerous drug" without being specially registered with the Bureau of Narcotics and Dangerous Drugs—then he or she is a "pusher" and must be severely punished, perhaps by life imprisonment.

Although it was obvious at the time of the witch hunts that the inquisitors profited handsomely from ferreting out and persecuting witches, neither this fact (no doubt too simple for the human mind craving complexity where none exists) nor the nonexistence of a witch problem before the thirteenth century was enough to help people realize what a horrible farce they were taking part in and witnessing. All this is even more dramatically true for today's horrible farce. Drug-abuseology—the creation of drug abusers and drug addicts and their persecution by means of "treatments"—is a flourishing business. In New York State alone, the state government has spent more than 6 billion dollars in the past half-dozen years[10]—not counting federal funds—with the wholly predictable result that the "drug problem" is now said to be worse than it has ever been. In the nineteenth century, when there were no drug controls, there was no drug problem.

The people—as the Grand Inquisitor so well understood—love being entertained and terrorized by campaigns to "save" them from "enemies," and are eager to embrace their leaders for offering to lift the burden of freedom from their shoulders. In each case, of course, the people were told—and felt that they had no "reason" to doubt that it was so—that their leaders were only protecting them, from witches and pushers, and were saving them, for God and Health. (See Table 1.)

Under the weight of a ceaseless egalitarian and anti-capitalist propaganda (in Communist and non-Communist countries alike) and the pressure of incessant programs of "drug education," most people have come to trust the unselfish State and to distrust those who "profit" from the sale and use of "dangerous drugs." All this make it easy for the Medical Inquisition gradually to escalate both the intensity and the range of its operations, without incurring serious opposition either from the popular press or from professional groups. No "serious" opinion makers protested early, when the first lies about "narcotics" were enshrined as official truths and when civil rights were first brushed aside by zealous prohibitionists fresh out of a job.

Long before the current dual "final solutions" for heroin addiction—that is, mandated methadone for the addicts and life imprisonment for the pushers—were proposed, there were a number of weapons introduced into the war against drugcraft that left no doubt about where this campaign was heading. Physicians or their surrogates were surreptitiously testing for illegal drugs in blood and urine—taken mainly from children, servicemen, and mental hospital patients. There was no protest. Persons and cars, stopped by law officers for reasons unrelated to drugs, were searched and, if drugs were found, the people were prosecuted for

TABLE 1
THE THEOCRATIC AND THERAPEUTIC
PERSPECTIVES IN SUMMARY

	THEOCRATIC STATE	THERAPEUTIC STATE
Dominant Ideology	Religious/Christian	Scientific/medical
Dominant value	Grace	Health
Interpreters, justifiers, prescribers, and proscribers of conduct and their ostensible aim	Priests Clerics Nuns Saving souls	Physicians Clinicians Nurses Curing bodies and minds
Heroes	Saints	Heroic healers
Heretics	Witches	Quacks
Ceremonies and Rituals	Baptism Holy Eucharist Confession, penance Holy Orders Holy Matrimony Miracles Exorcism Extreme Unction	Medical birth certification Psychopharmacology Psychotherapy M.D. degree Psychiatry as medical specialty Transplants Electroshock, lobotomy Medical death certification
Panaceas	Faith Hope Charity Holy water	Scientific knowledge Scientific research Compulsory treatment Therapeutic drugs
Panapathogens	Satan Blasphemy Witch's brew Jews and Jewish poisoners	Christian Scientists and others who defy the authority of medicine Rejection of medical science and medical treatment "Dangerous drugs" Drug addicts and pushers
Prohibited objects	The Bible in the "vulgar" tongue "Dangerous books" (Index of prohibited books)	Drugs in the free market "Dangerous drugs" (Index of prohibited drugs)
Unprofessional conduct	Selling too many indulgences Questioning the infallibility of the Mother Church	Writing too many prescriptions for "dangerous drugs" Questioning the infallibility of modern medicine
Agency of social sanction	The Inquisition	Institutional psychiatry
Aim of social sanction	Forced religious conversion	Forced psychiatric personality change
Intended domain or sphere of influence	The world	The world

violating anti-drug laws. There was no protest. In the late 1960s, many communities in New York State initiated a new "program" to "solve" the drug problem. Called TIP, it consisted of offering a monetary reward to anyone who would "turn in a pusher." So was the ancient art of denouncing one's friends, neighbors, and enemies to the authorities—in the public interest, to be sure—rediscovered in the Empire State. And there was no protest.

The more brazen and bizarre the methods of the persecutors became, the more enthusiastically were the persecutions embraced—as the unselfish acts of "concerned" public servants. Colleges had visiting lecturers talk about drug abuse and drug control. Medical schools mounted "crash programs" in drug abuse and its treatment. Most people—laymen and professionals—agreed with all that the authorities told them. Some knew better but kept their peace, fearing, usually rightly, for their own position, good name, and financial security. A few voiced dissent, generally to be ignored.

To be sure, there were many who complained and disagreed. But, just as it happened during the escalating terrors of other crusades, mass movements, and revolutions, nearly all who complained, and who complained the most self-righteously, complained about the wrong thing—strengthening, rather than weakening, the basic intellectual and moral premises of the persecutors. This is exemplified by those who now protest against mandatory life sentences for drug pushers as "excessive," losing sight of the fundamental moral and legal illegitimacy of punishing "pushers" at all! Many people are shocked at the idea that pushers should not be punished at all. Their reaction to this suggestion is much like that of people after the Inquisition and the Nazi program were well established: there could be no question then—even in the minds of the most "liberal" and "well-meaning" persons—that "something had to be done" with or to witches and Jews. "Reasonable" people could debate only what that "something" ought to be. The suggestion that nothing should be done would, in the first two instances, have constituted heresy and anti-Nazism; and would, in the third instance, be viewed as advocating the heroinization of helpless children from Harlem to Honolulu.

Perhaps it is necessary for such "crowd madnesses"[11] to run their course, and for masses of people to be injured, before enough people turn on them and reject them.

On February 2, 1973, *The New York Times* printed one of its countless reports on the war on drugcraft. Of course, it wasn't called that. It was entitled "Governor's Plan on Drug Abuse."[12] It occupied the better part of a whole page. The similarities between this program, which I shall review, and the programs of the witch hunters of a few hundred years ago will be apparent.

The report opens with this sentence: "Governor Rockefeller's proposals for dealing with drug traffickers have thus far dominated the 1973 Legislature, which completed its fifth work week today."[13] Here the main business of the Medical Inquisition is identified: the pushers "responsible" for the calamity of drug-craft.

"The Governor's proposals grew in large measure out of his frustration at the *failure* [my emphasis] of one of his own creations—the Narcotics Addiction Control Commission—to stem the narcotics epidemic."[14]

The word "failure" is significant here, for it expresses, in highly condensed form, the whole ideology of the war on drugcraft: the authorities who create the "problem" claim that they try to "solve" it but "fail." But if one rejects this ideology and mythology, then one would have to say that Governor Rockefeller's "creation" was not a dismal failure, but a huge success: it succeeded in still further exacerbating the "problem" it ostensibly set out to remedy. The authorities, however, now define addiction mongering as the opposite of what it actually is—just as they did formerly with witch mongering. And, because they *are* the authorities, they can impose their definition on the press and the popular mind. The correspondent for the *Times* seems to acknowledge this, in ending his report with this telling sentence: "But there is general agreement that whatever hard-line bill finally emerges will bear the Governor's imprimatur since he, by dint of his office and the huge public-relations apparatus at his command, brought and is still bringing intense attention to the issue."[15]

" 'Treatment alone [the *Times* report continues] cannot stop the spread of hard drugs and the gradual destruction of our society,' Mr. Rockefeller told the legislative hearing. What is needed now, he said, 'is a truly effective deterrent to the pushing of drugs.' "[16] In this view, the premise that "pushers" are bad people and that they are somehow "responsible" not only for the use of hard drugs but also for "the destruction of our society" is no longer debatable. Nor was Governor Rockefeller deterred from offering this suggestion by the fact that, only a few weeks earlier, the New York City Police Department was exposed in the press as having "pushed"—or should one say "lost"?—many million dollars' worth of heroin and cocaine.[17]

"Mr. Rockefeller has asked for mandatory life sentences for hard-drug dealers and for drug pushers who commit violent crimes. . . . The Governor has asked that the state pay bounties of $1,000 to persons who inform on a pusher who is convicted. . . . Hard drugs are defined in the legislation as heroin, cocaine, morphine, opium, hashish, LSD, and amphetamines. Marijuana is not included."[18]

The drama of the competition between accredited and non-accredited tempters (priests, healers, drug dealers, etc.) is here writ large: those who tempt others by offering them illegal drugs for sale are condemned and vilified as "pushers"; whereas those who tempt heroin addicts to become methadone addicts by offering them free methadone, who tempt informers to denounce people as addicts by offering them bounties, and who tempt doctors to prostitute themselves as state-salaried addiction mongers—all these are exalted and deified as "therapists" and as selfless fighters in the "war against drug abuse."

What criticism there has been against these proposals has centered entirely, as I remarked earlier, on the "excessive severity" of some of the penalties. Thus, some critics have warned that such harsh punishments might "encourage an addict to shoot a witness and might thus impose additional hazards on victims of addicts. 'This is a risk,' the Governor said recently."[19]

Other objections have been similarly feeble and indeed pitiful. "Some lawyers and legislators feel," the *Times* report continues, that "this [the bounty] would encourage dishonest and vindictive individuals to plant narcotics on people, opening up the possibility of innocent people being sentenced for life."[20]

This passage reveals that Americans—even lawyers and legislators!—have now fully accepted that they should not have a right to buy and sell certain drugs. If a people want to strip themselves of a right—which they possessed prior to 1914 and whose loss they do not even feel, much less understand—they will surely do so. One cannot make another person free, much less a whole nation. But it then remains for that nation to face the consequences of its decision: It must henceforth punish those who wish to exercise these "illegal" freedoms; it must reconcile its anti-capitalistic fervor with respect to drugs with its otherwise still capitalistic ideologies and institutions; and it must live with itself—which societies no less than individuals must be able to do—in the wee hours of the morning when it must realize that it savagely persecutes pushers, who like the abortionists of such recent past, merely offer a product or service for which there is an intense demand, while it indecisively indulges those who commit countless acts of direct violence against their fellow citizens.

Many authorities, of course, hail every new intensification of the battle as a welcome step "forward," and urge an even further escalation of weaponry. Thus, an editorial in the *Syracuse Herald-Journal* not only endorses everything that Rockefeller proposes, but complains that "those plans are for the pushers. What about those who turn a neat profit out of the drug traffic's byproducts, we wonder? Aren't those who sell the accessories, water pipes, cocaine spoons, hash pipes, rollers of marijuana joints, as guilty at least as any other individual convicted of contributing to the delinquency of a minor? . . . Sleazy profit-taking, isn't it?"[21]

On February 5, 1973, the New York State Conservative Party outbid Governor Rockefeller in its fervor in waging the holy war against drugcraft: while the Party recommended that the life sentence be "available" rather than mandatory for "street dealers," it also recommended the death penalty for "major importers and wholesalers of illicit drugs."[22] It is only fitting that as formerly the most faithful Christians favored the most un-Christian ferocity against witches, so now the most faithful capitalists recommend the most anti-capitalist ferocity against the entrepreneurs who trade in "dangerous drugs."

The popes convinced the people that witches were the transcendent malefactors of their society, and that they therefore deserved merciless punishment. The politicians have similarly convinced the people that drug pushers are the transcendent malefactors of our society, and that they therefore deserve merciless punishment. What the people did not realize then was that *they* were the witches and the bewitched, and what they do not realize now is that *they* are the pushers and the addicts. With monotonous regularity, the people foolishly fear the harmless scapegoats, and blindly trust the dangerous scapegoaters.

6. OPIUM AND ORIENTALS: THE MODEL AMERICAN SCAPEGOATS

As the scientific revolution displaced the religious ideology with a medical one, so the technological revolution, which it engendered, displaced human labor with the "work" of the machine. This transformation too had an immense influence on personal patterns of drug use and on cultural reactions to it. Until the advent of the machine, most men had to labor most of the time to survive. Hence, most of the major drugs that affect behavior—in particular, marijuana, opium, and cocaine—were used to enable men to work better, harder, and longer. These drugs were to pretechnological man what machines are to technological man: they helped him to increase "productivity" or "output." These facts have, of course, been brushed aside—indeed, they have been denied and falsified—by the evangelists of our modern pharmacomythologies.

By the middle of the nineteenth century, human labor was a glut on the market. In the relatively free market economies then prevailing, this meant that those who labored the hardest were at an advantage vis-à-vis their less productive competitors. Thus we enter the stage of modern history where we witness the most brutal wars of exclusion and extermination waged by the less gifted and industrious against those more so.

White Americans came in contact with and had to compete with three major racial groups whose habits differed fundamentally from their own: the native Indians, the African Negroes, and the Orientals—first chiefly the Chinese, then the Japanese. For reasons obvious to the contemporary reader, the Indians and Negroes could not—except in a few fields—hold their own or excel against the white Americans. Hence, they were demeaned as lazy and stupid—the degenerate members of inferior races. White Americans found their first match in the Chinese. The way they dealt with him is essential for our understanding of our "drug problem."

Chinese began to arrive in the United States in large numbers after 1850. Soon they outperformed and outproduced all the other races and nationalities, in the laundries and on the farms, in the mines and on the railroad. How did they do it? I cannot answer this question any better than anyone else can. I can only point to two facts—one obvious, the other not—that bear on the explanation: tradition and opium. The Chinese have always been regarded as intelligent, industrious, and well-disciplined. They also used opium, mainly by smoking it, much as Americans smoked tobacco. If the opium did not help them work better—although most of those who smoked it claimed that it did—it evidently did not hinder them! If white Americans had thought that it hindered them, they would have encouraged, or at least permitted, their use of opium, as they permitted and encouraged the use of alcohol among the Indians and Eskimos. As we shall see, this is not what happened. Instead, the Americans tried to exclude the Chinese so they would not have to compete with them, and tried to handicap them as competitors by depriving them of opium, whose habitual but moderate use helped them to cope with life and its vicissitudes. The persecution of the Chinese, between approximately 1880 and the First World War, forms one of the most instructive chapters in the history, not only of the United States, but also of drug use and psychiatry. I shall cite only the most salient facts of this story.

From the beginning, the anti-Chinese movement in America was led by the labor unions, first by those on the west coast, then by the national unions. Mainly as a result of their efforts, Congress enacted, in 1889, the Chinese Exclusion Act, barring the further immigration of Chinese into the United States.[1] This law, of course, had no effect on the approximately 100,000 Chinese left in the United States. Anti-Chinese agitation was henceforth directed against this group. In the course of this war against an exceptionally hard-working and law-abiding people, their characteristic habit—smoking opium—became the leading symbol of their "dangerousness." After all, Americans could not admit that they hated and feared the Chinese because the Chinese worked harder and were willing to work for lower wages than they did; they could no more do this than the Germans could admit that they hated and feared the Jews because the Jews worked harder and were more thrifty than they were. In each case—in all such cases

—a less competent majority attributes an evil to a more competent minority which then justifies the former in persecuting the latter.

That such charges are false; that, in fact, they are usually what psychiatrists call "projections"—the attributions of qualities lacking in the victims but very much present in the victimizers—makes this tactic all the more useful. For we must remember that this strategy can be used only by a powerful and vocal majority against a powerless and voiceless minority—which is what makes it work so well. The majority *defines* what the scapegoated minority is like, and *imposes* that definition on him. Americans thus defamed not only the Chinese but opium as well. Significantly, while no educated person still believes the ugly nonsense heaped on the Chinese for decades by leading American authorities, most educated persons still believe the ugly nonsense heaped on opium. The amazing success of this anti-opium campaign is revealed by juxtaposing two authoritative American opinions on this drug, one expressed in 1915, the other in 1970.

In 1915, the lead sentence in a lead article in the *Journal of the American Medical Association* characterized opium thus: "If the entire materia medica at our disposal were limited to the choice and use of only one drug, I am sure that a great many, if not the majority, of us would choose opium; and I am convinced that if we were to select, say half a dozen of the most important drugs in the Pharmakopeia, we should all place opium in the first rank."[2]

In 1970, at a United Nations conference called to enact new anti-drug treaties, the Director of the United States Bureau of Narcotics and Dangerous Drugs, acting as the chief U.S. delegate to the conference, offered this view on opium: "The social consequences of continuing opium production far exceed the medical or economic advantages of having it available. Halfway measures will not suffice—only total worldwide prohibition as soon as possible can eliminate this scourge of mankind."[3]

The pharmacological effects of *opium* have not changed between 1915 and 1970. It is clear what has: official and popular American *opinion* about opium.

Some further facts concerning the anti-Chinese movement will show not only the stereotyped pattern of such persecutions but also its close connection to the transformation of opium from a panacea (cure-all) to a panapathogen ("cause-all" of disease).[4]

At its first meeting in 1881, the first act of the Federation of Organized Trades and Labor Unions was to condemn the Chinese cigarmakers of California and to urge that only union-label cigars be bought. Nor were the leaders of the Federation, which became the American Federation of Labor in 1886, content merely to sanction the movement against the Chinese. They became, writes Herbert Hill, "the most articulate champions of the anti-Oriental cause in America."[5] The general who led this war of the American workingman against the Chinese coolie was Samuel Gompers, the president of the American Federation of Labor except for a single year, from its founding in 1886 until his death in 1924. Although himself an immigrant Jew who espoused socialist ideals and spouted the rhetoric of the solidarity of the toiling masses, he became a major spokesman in America for concepts of racial superiority, especially in labor.

In 1902 Gompers published a pamphlet, co-authored with Herman Gutstadt, another official of the A.F.L., entitled *Some Reasons for Chinese Exclusion: Meat vs. Rice, American Manhood Against Asiatic Coolieism—Which Shall Survive?* The pamphlet was written at the behest of the Chinese Exclusion Convention of 1901, its purpose being to persuade Congress to renew the Act, which was due to expire the following year. (It was renewed.) In this document, Gompers declares that "the racial differences between American whites and Asiatics would never be overcome. The superior whites had to exclude the inferior Asiatics by law, or if necessary, by force of arms. . . . The Yellow Man found it natural to lie, cheat, and murder and 99 out of every 100 Chinese are gamblers."[6]

Gompers never tired of repeating these racist lies, embellishing them, as I shall presently show, with the threat of opium. In 1906, for example, he intones that the "maintenance of the nation depended upon maintenance of racial purity";[7] and he pleads that it is contrary to "national interest" to allow the immigration of "cheap labor that could not be Americanized and could not be taught to render the same intelligent efficient service as was supplied by American workers."[8]

Presaging by many decades the press-agentry of totalitarian propagandists, Gompers creates, out of his hate-filled fantasies, the image of the Chinese opium fiend—an image whose impact has possibly been even greater than the impact of the famous Nazi mendacities. According to Hill, "Gompers conjures up a terrible picture of how the Chinese entice little white boys and girls into becoming 'opium fiends.' Condemned to spend their days in the back of laundry rooms, these tiny lost souls would yield up their virgin bodies to their maniacal yellow captors. 'What other crimes were committed in those dark fetid places,' Gompers writes, 'when these little innocent victims of the Chinamen's viles were under the influence of the drug, are almost too horrible to imagine. . . . There are hundreds, aye, thousands, of our American girls and boys who have acquired this deathly habit and are doomed, hopelessly doomed, beyond the shadow of redemption.' "[9]

Nixon and McGovern, Rockefeller and Lindsay, the officials of the American Medical Association and the American Bar Association, all the guardians of our morals and health regardless of party or profession, now repeat this anti-Chinese fantasy about opium as if it were the Gospel. Because it is "gospel." The tempter —Chinaman, Turkish farmer, or American "pusher"—is the devil in whose grip the pure, innocent American is entangled as helplessly as a fly in a spider's web. Not a pretty picture, this—whether one believes it, and is thereby urged to commit the most awful acts justified by visions of "therapy"; or whether one disbelieves it, and is therefore driven to the most uncompromising rejection of authorities so bereft of common sense and common decency.

That the early American anti-opium attitudes were initiated by racial rather than medical considerations is the inescapable lesson that this story teaches us. Even the Consumers Union Report on *Licit and Illicit Drugs,* which is strongly prejudiced against drugs —especially opiates—acknowledges this fact. The following passages from the Report support this contention, and also reveal that the anti-Chinese persecution in America was directed not only against the Chinaman as a human being but also against his characteristic habit—a habit that was a part of his "life style" and which enabled him to be "whole," to be effective, and to outperform the white American.

"To summarize the data reviewed so far," write Edward M. Brecher and his collaborators, "opiates taken daily in large doses . . . were not a social menace under nineteenth-century conditions, and were not perceived as a menace . . . and there was little demand for opiate prohibition. But there was one exception to this general tolerance of the opiates. In 1875, the City of San Francisco [which even then was 'wide open'] adopted an ordinance prohibiting the smoking of opium in smoking houses or 'dens.' The roots of this ordinance were racist rather than health-oriented. . . ."[10]

These and other similar prohibitions failed to stop the use of opium; instead, according to contemporary observers, they "seemed to add zest to [its] enjoyment."[11] Soon Congress stepped in and, in 1887, enacted a law prohibiting the importation of opium by the Chinese, but not by Americans! In 1890, a law was passed that restricted the manufacture of smoking opium to American citizens![12] In 1909, the importation of smoking opium was prohibited altogether. Henceforth, the opiates used and "abused" were morphine and heroin—habits in which the Chinese had no further interest.

The American war against the Chinese in the United States was a terrible tragedy—regardless of how often this drama continues to be enacted on the stage of history. Although "we" did not succeed in beating "them" down, at least "we" took away something that "they" treasured and that made life better for "them." Envious persecutors must be thankful for small victories no less than for large. The Turks were more successful in their war against the Armenians; the Germans in theirs against the Jews; and the Ugandans in theirs against the East Indians. Each of these wars was, I submit, fueled largely—if not wholly—by the envy of an inferior majority directed against a superior minority.[13] This is the scenario: the majority redefines the minority as inferior and debased—and hence a danger to its own "purity"; and, having thus concealed and justified its aggressive aims against its successful competitor, the majority rids itself of its "pollutant"—by expelling or eradicating the minority.

While this war against the Chinese and their opium habit—which was to have such amazingly far-reaching consequences a century later!—was taking place in the United States, countless other persons were using drugs which are now illegal, especially opium and cocaine, in an effort to help them cope with the demands of life. Among these persons were two world-famous physicians. Their use of "dangerous drugs" provides as dramatic a refutation of the contemporary "scientific" claims concerning the effects of these drugs as one could imagine. Both of these men used drugs to enable them to fulfill their ambitions to succeed—and to succeed in medicine, at that!

One of these doctors was Sigmund Freud (1856–1939). The drug he used was cocaine. The story, set forth in Ernest Jones's *Life and Work of Sigmund Freud,* is briefly as follows:

"I have been reading about cocaine, the essential ingredient of coca leaves, which some Indian tribes chew to enable them to resist privations and hardships," writes Freud to his fiancée, Martha Bernays, on April 21, 1884.[14] Freud then tries cocaine in small doses and finds that it relieves his depression without robbing him of any energy for work. On May 25, 1884, he writes to Martha Bernays: "If it goes well I will write an essay on it and I expect it will win its place in therapeutics side by side with morphine and superior to it. I have other hopes and intentions about it. I take very small doses of it regularly against indigestion, and with the most brilliant success."[15]

In July 1884 Freud publishes his essay on cocaine, in which he reviews the literature on the subject and reports on his own experiences with the drug, which Jones summarizes as follows: "He wrote of the 'exhilaration and lasting euphoria, which in no way differs from the normal euphoria of the healthy person. . . . You perceive an increase of self-control and possess more vitality and capacity for work. . . . In other words, you are simply normal, and it is soon hard to believe that you are under the influence of any drug. . . . Long intensive mental or physical work is performed without any fatigue. . . . This result is enjoyed without any of the unpleasant aftereffects that follow exhilaration brought about by alcohol.' "[16]

In this essay, Freud recommends the use of cocaine for the treatment of "neurasthenia." He himself uses the drug for three years, after which he gives it up without any difficulty.

This story hardly requires comment. I would like to remark only that Freud used cocaine in two distinct, but psychologically closely related, ways—a distinction that has been remarkably neglected in the literature on psychoactive drugs. First, he used the drug on himself, to bolster his energy in the service of his boundless ambition to leave his mark on the world. Second, he used the drug on patients and made extravagant claims for his therapeutic success with it. In short, cocaine made him a stronger man and a more effective doctor. When he found other ways of being strong and effective—as a person and as a therapist—he gave up this particular method of coping with stress. The answer to whether a person finds it easy or difficult to give up a drug habit thus lies not in the drug, but in the use to which the person who takes it puts it, and in the substitutes for it that he can or wants to employ.

It is interesting to note here that Freud's work with, and use of, cocaine evidently embarrassed his reverential biographer, Jones. Indeed, perhaps it is precisely because Freud himself was a cocaine "addict" in the present-day sense of this term, and because he was also "addicted" to cigars, that psychoanalysts have put forward such peculiar and plainly misleading views on addiction— the most revealing being that Freud was simply not an addict at all. His use of cocaine is discounted by Jones with the phrase "the cocaine episode," and with this remarkable reassertion of the master's "mental health": ". . . as we now know, it needs a special disposition to develop a drug addiction, and fortunately Freud did not possess that."[17] In exactly the same way, neither Jones nor other "orthodox" psychoanalysts consider or classify Freud's smoking as an addiction. On the contrary, Freud's cigar, like his couch, became a significant symbol of the psychoanalyst's professional identity.

These two habits of Freud's, and their interpretation by respected psychiatric historians and psychoanalytic theoreticians, should, in my opinion, command our closest attention. For, to repeat, when the founder of psychoanalysis gives up cocaine after using it for three years, his followers cite this as evidence of his mental health! And when Freud smokes cigars immoderately and cannot function without them, that prompts them to incorporate cigars into the ceremonial chemistry of the psychoanalytic ritual! Perhaps Freud could give up cocaine but not cigars because he could feel that he was "himself" without cocaine in his body, but that he was not "himself" without a cigar in his mouth.

When people find that a drug which they use to cope with life as they want to cope with it hinders rather than helps them, they then give up using that drug and give it up easily. Since the kind of "coping" we are considering here is often a matter of gaining superiority over people, we would expect that almost anything that helps a person—especially if he has a powerful urge to dominate or excel—to control others or surpass them, would help him to relinquish certain drug habits; and similarly, that almost anything that helps him to put others down—to render them inferior, subservient, or stigmatized—would also help him to do so. This interpretation is consistent not only with the fact that "drug addiction" is common among young people who often give up their habit as they grow older, but also with the life histories of many famous drug users, for example, Freud and Malcolm X,[18] each of whom easily relinquished his particular, socially disapproved drug habit as he developed his distinctive, socially approved work habit with which he was able to imprint his mark on the world—the one through the psychoanalytic movement, and the other through the Black Power movement.

The case of another famous physician who had been addicted to the "hardest" of "hard" drugs, morphine, shows that even this drug may, depending on the subject's abilities and motives, be used to help the "addict" to meet instead of to evade his responsibilities.

Dr. William Stewart Halsted (1852–1922), one of the greatest and most famous American surgeons and a founder of the Johns Hopkins medical school, was a lifelong morphine addict. Shortly after entering private practice in New York in the 1870s, Halsted became addicted to cocaine, a habit he could break only by be-coming a morphine addict. Thus, when, in 1886, Dr. William Henry Welch invited Halsted to join the group that founded the Johns Hopkins medical school, Halsted, then thirty-four, was a morphine addict. This information became available only in 1969, when, on the occasion of the eightieth anniversary of the opening of the Johns Hopkins Hospital, the "secret history" of the Hopkins, written by another of its founders, Sir William Osler, was made public. "When we recommended him as full surgeon," wrote Osler in that document, ". . . I believed, and Welch did too, that he was no longer addicted to morphine. He had worked so well and so energetically that it did not seem possible that he could take the drug and do so much."[19]

Actually, it was not despite his use of morphine but because of it that Halsted could do so much. After Osler gained his confidence, he learned that "[Halsted] had never been able to reduce the amount to less than three grains [180 milligrams] daily; on this he could do his work comfortably and maintain his excellent physical vigor . . . I do not think that anyone suspected him, not even Welch."[20]

While on morphine, "Halsted married into a distinguished Southern family; his wife had been head nurse in the operating rooms at the Hopkins. They lived together in 'complete mutual devotion' until Halsted's death thirty-two years later."[21] In 1898, at the age of forty-six, Halsted reduced his daily dose of morphine to a grain and a half [90 milligrams]. According to Edward Brecher, "he remained in good health, active, esteemed, and in all probability addicted, until the end."[22]

Perhaps it is time now to add to one of the legendary quips about the Hopkins. When the entrance standards for the Johns Hopkins medical school were established, Sir William Osler remarked to Dr. William H. Welch: "Welch, it is lucky that we get in as professors; we could never enter as students."[23] If these venerable physicians are now in their well-deserved heavenly resting place, we might imagine Dr. Halsted saying to Dr. Welch: "Welch, it is lucky that you had let me in as a professor; now you would let me in only as a patient at the Phipps [the psychiatric division of the Johns Hopkins Hospital], with the diagnosis of 'personality disorder: morphine addiction.' "

The foregoing evidence clearly justifies the conclusion that addictions are habits; that habits enable us to do some things, and disable us from doing others; and hence, that we may, indeed must, judge addictions as good or bad according to the value we place on what they enable us to do or disable us from doing. Furthermore, what any particular habit enables a person to do, or disables him from doing, may—as we have seen—be either a matter of fact or a matter of attribution. Although this is obvious, it must be re-emphasized because of the ever-present human tendency—now directed especially toward certain pharmacological agents—to make utterly false attributions of harmfulness to scapegoats. (There is a similar tendency to make false attributions of helpfulness to panaceas, which I shall consider later.)[24]

All this points to the all-too-familiar powers of authority to define what is good and what is bad, and hence social reality itself. I should like to apply this principle to addictions as enabling and disabling habits, by briefly re-examining the parable of the Fall as an example of the acquisition of an "addiction."

According to the Judeo-Christian mythology of creation, the first "bad" habit which man and woman acquired was making moral judgments. Having eaten the forbidden fruit, usually identified as an apple, Adam and Eve "realize" that they are naked and cover their genital organs. Henceforth, they—like God!—make moral judgments of what is good and evil, of what pleases and displeases them. They are thus subject to pain and suffering, but also experience pleasure and the love of life. They copulate and enjoy it, but how could they enjoy it if they did not also feel desire and frustration?

Original sin thus engenders the "original habit" which enable Adam and Eve to do some things they could not do before acquiring it. Specifically, through eating the Apple, Adam and Eve became strong enough to live an independent and free existence, quite unlike the indolent life to which God made them accustomed in the Garden of Eden. Like the South American Indian's coca leaves or, not so long ago, the North American housewife's opium,[25] the Apple makes it possible for man and woman to endure life and fulfill their domestic duties. Truly, the Apple—the Forbidden Fruit—is man's first encounter with an "illegal" or "prohibited" drug; eating it helps him to cope with life, not to cop out as he had done before eating it.

Moreover, to uphold His authority in forbidding the Fruit, God evidently feels justified in lying to man. Man's liberation from bondage to authority thus begins with two simultaneous acts: defiance of a prohibition—eating the Apple; and calling God's bluff—unmasking the Divine Deception.

By Divine Deception I refer to God's initial exposition of His rules governing man's conduct: "The Lord God took the man and put him in the garden of Eden to till and keep it. And the Lord God commanded the man, saying, 'You may freely eat of every tree of the garden; but of the tree of the knowledge of good and evil you shall not eat, for in the day that you eat of it you shall die.' "[26] The Serpent counsels Eve to eat the Fruit, explicitly exhorting her as follows: " 'You will not die. For God knows that when you eat of it your eyes will be opened, and you will be like God, knowing good and evil.' "[27]

In short, God lies to man, whereas the Serpent tells him the truth. There is a hint here of a profound insight into the relationship between power and deceit, and independence and candor. To maintain his domination over his subject, authority will resort to both force and fraud. In contrast, he who lacks the power to oppress but possesses instead independence—a gift neither the superior nor the subordinate enjoys, as each depends on the other—can afford the luxury of seeing and saying the truth.

The contention that God deceived man—that He threatened that the consequence of eating the Fruit was death when actually it was life—is borne out not only by the fact that Adam and Eve did not perish after their trespass, but also by the whole new set of punishments which God metes out to the culprits: He curses the Serpent and makes him crawl on his belly; He makes childbearing painful, and woman subordinate to man; He sentences man to a life of unremitting labor; and He makes man and woman mortal![28]

In Theocratic Societies, authorities have used God and Religion to bully man into submission; in Therapeutic Societies, they use Science and Medicine to do so. And, just as formerly God and the priests have deceived man, so, I submit, Science and the physicians deceive him now. "Eat the Fruit and you will die!" God had warned, but it wasn't true. "Use the Drug, and you will become hooked, you will become bad and mad, and you will die!" Science now warns, but it isn't true. Only by defying God and unmasking the Divine Deception could our forebears overthrow the tyranny of God; only by defying Science and unmasking the Therapeutic Deception can modern man and woman overthrow the tyranny of Science. This defiance of deception—by God, Pope, King, the Majority, Science—has always been, and perhaps will always be, the highest duty of the individual.

7. DRUGS AND DEVILS: THE CONVERSION CURE OF MALCOLM X

Judging by the evidence of anthropologists, historians, and students of religion, most of mankind has been, and continues to be, bedazzled by the spectacle of human tragedy as a sort of cosmic recycling of vice into virtue, evil into good—and vice versa. As a result, the themes of pollution and purification, of vilification and glorification, and generally of devilification and deification, continue to exercise a hypnotic influence over individuals and groups.

In the past, the standard scenario for this drama was cast in the imagery of religion, and particularly of the Christian religion: the sinner was saved; the heathen, the Jew, the Mohammedan was converted to the true faith; the Messiah came to save mankind, and, in the end, after death, all were promised the possibility of redemption and salvation—and indeed a sort of immortal "life" as "dead men"—in a "life hereafter."

Today, the scenario for the same plot is medical and racial: the patient is cured; the homosexual becomes heterosexual; the alcoholic and addict become the ex-alcoholic and ex-addict; the fearful European Jew becomes the fearless Israeli; the timid housewife becomes the tough women's-libber; and the humble Negro becomes the proud Black Muslim.

In short, as in the Age of Faith the hero was the redeemed sinner, so in the Age of Madness and Racism the hero is the ex-addict and inverted racist. Among the major heroes of this type so characteristic of our age, and of our country, is Malcolm X.

The metamorphosis of Malcolm X from drug addict to revolutionary leader and assassinated saint epitomizes the theme of pollution and purification in the currently fashionable images and rhetoric of drugs and racism.

The front cover of the paperback edition of his *Autobiography* —which is the source of my following remarks—describes him in this way: "He rose from hoodlum, thief, dope peddler, pimp . . . to become the most dynamic leader of the Black Revolution."[1]

There are some remarkable parallels—which I only want to note here and shall not discuss further—between the lives of Jean Genet and Malcolm X, and especially between the magnificent *Saint Genet*[2] by Sartre and the moving *Autobiography* by Malcolm X. However, as a purification rite, the conversion of a neglected, abused, and uneducated French orphan into a great French writer, or of a man ashamed of his homosexuality into one who is proud of it, simply does not compare, in its dramatic appeal and impact, especially for Americans, with the conversion of an impulsive Negro hoodlum into a superbly self-disciplined Black Panther, of a pitiful drug addict and despicable dope pusher into a Muslim Minister with the dignity and self-control of a Stoic philosopher or Spartan general. It is this transformation and self-transformation whose progress I wish to trace.

From a horrifying childhood, Malcolm (Little) X grew into an eighth-grade dropout, a teen-age "hustler," and, before he was quite twenty-one, a convict with a ten-year sentence for armed burglary. In the years before his arrest and imprisonment, he smoked and sold marijuana, sniffed cocaine, procured, lived off white women, stole and robbed, nearly murdered and was in turn nearly murdered on countless occasions. He could not sink much lower—nor rise much higher.

He was saved by his conversion to Black Muslimism, and specifically by the leader of this movement, Elijah Muhammad. Alex Haley, to whom Malcolm X dictated his *Autobiography*, reports that before they actually started to work on the book, Malcolm wrote out a statement which he intended as the dedication for the book. It read: "This book I dedicate to the Honorable Elijah Muhammad, who found me here in America in the muck and mire of the filthiest civilization and society on this earth, and pulled me out, cleaned me up, and stood me on my feet, and made me the man I am today."[3] This purification, beautification, and cleansing is what most of the book is about. Since, in the end, not even Elijah Muhammad could measure up to Malcolm X's standards of purity, this dedication does not appear at the front of the book.

For some time before his imprisonment, Malcolm X used large

quantities of marijuana. He writes: "Shorty had originally introduced me to marijuana, and my consumption of it now astounded him."[4] He also "sniffed" cocaine; he does not say in what quantities. He remarks, however, that "I viewed narcotics as most people regard food. I wore my guns as today I wear a necktie. Deep down, I actually believed that after living as fully as humanly possible, one should then die violently."[5] The drugs and violence were, in short, his life style or religion. This was for him, at that time, the right way to live.

In February 1946, shortly before his twenty-first birthday, Malcolm X was arrested and sentenced to ten years' imprisonment. By that time, he says, he had sunk to "the very bottom of the American white man's society"; and he adds: "soon now, in prison, I found Allah and the religion of Islam and it completely transformed my life."[6]

But not right away. During the first months in prison, Malcolm X continued, as best he could, the style of life he had led on the outside. He used drugs and profanity as much as possible. The men in his cell block actually nicknamed him "Satan"—"because of my antireligious attitude."[7] As for drugs, he tells us that "with some money sent by Ella [his sister], I was finally able to buy stuff for better highs from guards in the prison. I got reefers, Nembutal, and benzedrine. Smuggling to prisoners was the guards' sideline; every prison's inmates know that's how guards make most of their living."[8]

Malcolm's initiation into the Black Muslim religion began with letters from his brother, Reginald. The crucial first step, he says— and I believe him—was this instruction: "Malcolm, don't eat any more pork, and don't smoke any more cigarettes. I'll show you how to get out of prison."[9] A few days later, when pork was served for the noon meal, Malcolm did not eat any—and he experienced his first "high" from abstinence and purification. "I hesitated with the platter in mid-air; then I passed it along to the inmate waiting next to me. He began serving himself; abruptly, he stopped. I remember him turning, looking surprised at me.

"I said to him, 'I don't eat pork.'

"The platter then kept on down the table.

"It was the funniest thing, the reaction, and the way that it spread. In prison, where so little breaks the monotonous routine, the smallest thing causes a commotion of talk. It was being mentioned all over the cell block by night that Satan didn't eat pork. It made me very proud, in some odd way. One of the universal images of the Negro, in prison and out, was that he couldn't do without pork. It made me feel good to see that my not eating it had especially startled the white convicts."[10]

Malcolm X had a burning passion to be noticed and admired, feared and respected. Before his imprisonment, he tried to achieve respect and recognition in the only ways he knew: by using drugs and selling them; by abusing white women; and by outright violence. These methods still have severe limitations in our society, especially in the hands of poor Negroes. In abstinence from pork Malcolm glimpsed a whole new repertoire of ways to impress and control others; and so he discovered self-control. Moreover, being the supremely ambitious and energetic man that he was, he not only discovered self-control, but cultivated it and became as good at it as Joe Louis had been at boxing. He out-self-disciplined everyone around him, including, in the end, Elijah Muhammad. This, probably, was one of the reasons why he was assassinated. I shall, however, confine myself here to Malcolm X's conversion from self-indulgent drug user to stoic Black Muslim.

The two next most crucial steps in Malcolm X's personal metamorphosis—which, of course, was not nearly as great a change in his moral values as it was in the social consequences of how he acted on them—were his discovery that the greatest joys of self-indulgence can come from self-denial, and that the greatest prop for one's self-esteem is to be able to degrade, vilify, and make a scapegoat out of one's fellow man. So, abruptly and apparently effortlessly, Malcolm stopped smoking cigarettes and using drugs, and ate no more pork. And, most importantly, he learned, from the Muslim religion, to which first his brother and then Elijah Muhammad himself had converted him, that "the white man is the devil."[11] This may sound silly, or serious. Malcolm X took it as the most literal and important truth he ever possessed. And he acted on it.

His conversion was now complete. He had thought that marijuana and cocaine and guns were good, and that he knew how to beat the white man with them at his own game. But he realized that he had been grievously mistaken. The youthful troublemaker had matured to the self-disciplined fanatic. He was no longer *possessed*—by the devil, drugs, uncontrollable passions. He had turned the tables on them all: Now it was he who was *in possession*—of himself, of "the truth," and of the self-righteousness that came from knowing that his hatred of the white man, previously justified on flimsy pretexts, rested firmly on the "fact" that Whitey was the devil.

"The very enormity of my previous life's guilt prepared me to accept the truth,"[12] he writes. Modesty was never one of Malcolm's faults, although he tried to conceal, and apparently thought he had succeeded in concealing, his power drive behind the standard political and religious rhetoric of selflessness and devotion to the collective—the Nation of Islam. The truth, he continues, can, however, be "received only by the sinner who knows and admits that he is guilty of having sinned much. . . . I do not now, and I did not then [when he first read about him] liken myself to Paul. But I do understand his experience."[13]

The conversion of the Christian notion of sin as a requirement for salvation into the medical notion of sickness as a requirement for cure—that is, for medical salvation and success in the world ruled by the religion of medicine—has portentous implications which we ignore at our own peril. If left unchecked, we have, in this ideological premise, an incitement, a seduction, for people to assume the sick role and to play it for all it's worth, if only to be redeemed from it by miraculous cures which then lead straight to positions of prestige and power. Sanctified by recoveries—from alcoholism, drug addiction, and obesity today, and from who knows what other diseases tomorrow—the ex-patient becomes the prophet and ruler who can at last dominate and exploit, and be admired and glorified, instead of persecuted and vilified.

Through the years, and especially following his release from prison after serving seven years of his ten-year sentence, Malcolm practiced the rituals of the Black Muslims, which place great emphasis on orderliness and cleanliness. This is his description of his morning washing-up routine: " 'In the name of Allah, I perform the ablution,' the Muslim said aloud before washing first the right hand, then the left hand. The teeth were thoroughly brushed, followed by three rinsings out of the mouth. The nostrils also were rinsed out thrice. A shower then completed the whole body's purification in readiness for prayer."[14]

If only they didn't hate the whites so much, and vice versa, Muslims and white Puritans of the cleanliness-is-next-to-godliness school would obviously get along just fine. The trouble is that each has found the devil and is sure who he is: the other.

Clearly, the Black Muslims were imitating the Puritans—the name is significant in this connection—and were simply appropriating the Puritan ethic as their own discovery. (Perhaps all oppressed individuals and groups do this when they want to use something that belongs to their "enemy.") Here is the way Malcolm X explains "the code" by which the Muslims are expected to live: "Any fornication was absolutely forbidden in the Nation of Islam. Any eating of the filthy pork or other injurious or unhealthy foods; any use of tobacco, alcohol, or narcotics. No Muslim who followed Elijah Muhammad could dance, gamble, date, attend movies, or sports, or take long vacations from work. Muslims slept no more than health required. Any domestic quarreling, any discourtesy, especially to women, was not allowed. No lying or stealing, and no insubordination to civil authority, except on the grounds of religious obligation."[15]

In short, the Muslim code contains some of the best precepts on self-reliance that have been articulated from the ancient Greeks to Emerson, and since; however, it has been fanaticized and made to serve the ultimate end, not of respect for self through respect for others, but of respect for self through the dehumanization of all who are not "black."

Before his meteoric rise to prominence in the Black Power movement, Malcolm X was a conscientious minister. He was frugal and in all ways abstinent. "As in the case of all the Nation's ministers, my living expenses were paid and I had some pocket money. Where once you couldn't have named anything

I wouldn't have done for money, now money was the last thing to cross my mind."[16]

Power is, however, a jealous mistress. "I had always been very careful to stay completely clear of any personal closeness with any of the Muslim sisters," Malcolm continues. "My total commitment to Islam demanded having no other interests, especially, I felt, no women. . . . Islam has very strict laws and teachings about women, the core of them being that the true nature of a man is to be strong, and a woman's true nature is to be weak, and . . . that he must control her if he expects to get her respect."[17]

Every world-view represents, perforce, the preferences of the group that articulates it and uses it to justify its supremacy. The traditional Western, Judeo-Christian view is thus the tactical theory of the white male: both its theology and its science proclaim and "prove" the superiority of the white man over the black, and of man over woman. *Mutatis mutandis,* when the black man undertakes to dominate the white man, he invents his own theological and scientific mythologies to explain his ideas and justify his intentions. And the women who desire to dominate the men do likewise.[18]

We may recall, in this connection, that the Scriptures had long been used to explain and justify both white and male supremacism. It is much less well known, indeed it has been remarkably well suppressed, that Benjamin Rush—one of the "fathers" not only of white America but also of Institutional Psychiatry—put forth a theory about why the Negro is black that nearly everyone today would consider bizarre, and perhaps many did even then. Interestingly, this theory—which I presented in full in *The Manufacture of Madness*[19]—resembles closely Elijah Muhammad's theory of why the white man is white.

The similarities between Rush's theory and Muhammad's—each ostensibly accounting for the creation of humanity, each aggrandizing his own race and diminishing that of the other, as congenitally leprous, in the one case, and as the devil in the other—are, perhaps, not so surprising after all. People abhor monotony and crave variety. But, as there are only so many ways men and women can sexually stimulate each other or themselves, there are only so many ways that men and women—white, black, yellow, or red—can glorify themselves and vilify others. Indeed, it is precisely because these ways are, actually, few in number that the study of anthropology and history shows such remarkably recurrent patterns in human behavior, both individual and collective. The French have a maxim for this: "The more things change, the more they remain the same." Perhaps here, too, lies one of the reasons why men not only forget history, but often positively refuse to acknowledge it. Craving and stubbornly searching for novelty in life, where—except in the natural sciences and technology—such novelty is the rarest of rarities, men do not remember history so that they can, to paraphrase Santayana, rediscover it while repeating it.

Benjamin Rush (1746–1813), one of the signers of the Declaration of Independence, was a physician and a self-declared abolitionist. "I love even the name of Africa," he wrote to Jeremy Belknap, "and never see a Negro slave or free man without emotions which I seldom feel in the same degree toward my unfortunate fellow creatures of a fairer complexion."[20] What, then, did Rush have against Negroes: only that they all suffered from leprosy! How did Rush know this? Medical science told him so. The black man, Rush insisted, suffers from "congenital leprosy . . . in so mild a form that excess pigmentation was its only symptom."[21] Since this was a congenital form of the disease, the Negro remained safe as a servant, but was declared unsafe, and hence taboo, as a sexual partner. In short, Rush maintained that God created man as white, and if he is black it's because he has leprosy. Rush did not even bother to consider skin colors other than white and black, and hence did not have to reconcile the Indian's red skin with his medical theory of creation.

Elijah Muhammad has discovered and teaches another theory of creation, startlingly similar to Rush's. M. S. Handler, presumably unaware of Rush's theory, goes out of his way, in his Introduction to *The Autobiography,* to register his surprise at the "absurdity" of this patently "anti-theory" of white creation. "Malcolm's exposition of his social ideas was clear and thoughtful," writes Handler, "if somewhat shocking to the white initiate, but most disconcerting in our talk was Malcolm's belief in Elijah

Muhammad's history of the origins of man, and in a genetic
theory devised to prove the superiority of black over white—a
theory stunning to me in its sheer absurdity."[22]
   This passage points to the heart of the problem of science *as*
religion: we believe "our" science as gospel truth, and reject
"theirs" (whoever "they" may be) as absurdities. Yet the "science"
our government and medical schools now teach about alcoholism
and drug abuse as "diseases," and the treatments they propose and
practice to cure them, are not a whit less absurd than Muhammad's,
or for that matter Rush's, theory.
   What, then, is this "absurd" black theory of creation? I shall
summarize it as much as I can in Malcolm's own words. "Elijah
Muhammad teaches his followers [in what he calls "Yacub's History"] that, first, the moon separated from the earth. Then, the
first humans, Original Man, were a black people. They founded the
Holy City of Mecca. Among this black race were twenty-four wise
scientists. One of the scientists, at odds with the rest, created the
especially strong black tribe of Shabazz, from which America's
Negroes, so-called, descended."[23]
   There then came a time when a child was born—his name was
Yacub—who grew up to be an especially brilliant scientist. He
discovered how to "breed races scientifically." However, because
of his overwhelming pride and disrespect of established authority,
he was at last exiled from Mecca to the island of Patmos. On Patmos, Yacub went to work creating—what had evidently been missing in the Muslim religion until that point—the devil. "Though he
was a black man, Mr. Yacub, embittered toward Allah now, decided, as revenge, to create upon the earth a devil race—a bleached
out, white race of people."[24]
   And this Mr. Yacub did. Six hundred years passed "before this
race of people returned to the mainland, among the natural black
people. Mr. Elijah Muhammad teaches his followers that within
six months' time, through telling lies that set the black men fighting among each other, this devil race had turned what had been
a peaceful heaven on earth into a hell . . ."[25]
   This story of creation does not end on this sad note. It continues
on to this Black Muslim version of the "last becoming the first."

"It was written that after Yacub's bleached white race had ruled the world for six thousand years—down to our time—the black original race would give birth to one whose wisdom, knowledge, and power would be infinite. . . . Elijah Muhammad teaches that the greatest and mightiest God who appeared on the earth was Master W. D. Fard."[26]

The ideas this legend must have inspired in Malcolm X are not hard to imagine. He claims that he believed quite literally in the satanicity of the white man. Whether he believed equally literally, or only slightly less so, in his own divinity is not very important, at least for our understanding of the so-called drug problem.

The Black Muslims have, as we have seen already, a clear and consistent policy on drugs: they believe in strict abstinence from all self-indulgent pleasures. In an important sense, then, it is quite misleading to speak of a Black Muslim approach to the "treatment" of the addict, for if a person is a Muslim he cannot be an addict, just as if he is an Orthodox Jew he cannot be a pork eater. It's as simple as that.

In other words, the Muslim perspective on drug use and drug avoidance, like mine, is moral and religious. This does not mean, of course, that, from this perspective, we come to all the same conclusions.

Malcolm's passion for honesty and truth surfaces in some interesting drug demythologizings—that is, in assertions that fly in the face of some current scientific and medical dogmas about "hard" or "dangerous" drugs and their "addictive" powers. "Some prospective Muslims," Malcolm remarks as if it were an unimportant aside, "found it more difficult to quit tobacco than others found quitting the dope habit."[27] One gathers that it makes not much difference to Muslims whether a man smokes tobacco or marijuana: they know that what counts is the habit of "self-indulgence," not the pharmacomythology of "highs" or "kicks." Obviously one good mythology per person is enough: if you believe—really believe—in the mythology of Black Muslimism, or Judaism, or Christianity, then you don't need the ersatz mythology of Medicalism and Therapeutism.

The Muslims emphasize not only that addiction is evil but that,

like all the evil in the world except perhaps even more so, it is
one that is deliberately imposed on the Negro by the white man.
"The Muslim program began with recognizing that color and addiction have a distinct connection. It is no accident that in the
entire Western Hemisphere, the greatest localized concentration
of addicts is in Harlem."[28] The "monkey" on the addict's back is,
in the Muslim reality, Whitey. "Every addict," explains Malcolm,
"takes junk to escape something . . . most black junkies really
are trying to narcotize themselves against being a black man in
the white man's America. But, actually, the Muslim says, the black
man taking dope is only helping the white man to 'prove' that the
black man is nothing."[29]

This converts the struggle against the temptation of the drug
into a veritable struggle for "national liberation" from white oppression: it politicizes a personal problem, neatly reversing the
psychiatric tactic of personalizing political problems by declaring
embarrassing dissidents insane. (In my opinion, both are tactics,
and *nothing but* tactics.)

Muslims thus believe in breaking the drug habit by having the
addict go "cold turkey"—which means abrupt and complete withdrawal from the drug, the addict having to bear the suffering associated with this process. This ordeal actually helps further to
dramatize and ritualize the addict's liberation from Whitey. "When
the addict's withdrawal sets in," writes Malcolm, "and he is
screaming, cursing, and begging, 'Just one shot, man!' the Muslims are right there talking junkie jargon to him. 'Baby, knock
that monkey off your back! Kick that habit! Kick Whitey off your
back! . . . Let Whitey go, baby!' "[30]

Actually, the Black Muslims now say exactly what white physicians said fifty years ago—namely, that drug addiction is not a
disease, but a form of behavior of which they disapprove. Writing
in 1921 in the *Journal of the American Medical Association,*
here is how Alfred C. Prentice, M.D., a member of the Committee
on Narcotic Drugs of the American Medical Association, articulated the then "official" view on addiction: "Public opinion regarding the vice of drug addiction has been deliberately and
consistently corrupted through propaganda in both the medical

and lay press. . . . The shallow pretense that drug addiction is a 'disease' . . . has been asserted and urged in volumes of 'literature' by self-styled 'specialists.' "[31] Thus, the Muslims now support the same values, and conduct themselves in much the same way, as doctors did then; whereas both physicians and their black "patients" on methadone now cultivate the modes and manners of the "counter-culture."

Malcolm X wore his hair crew-cut, dressed with the severe simplicity and elegance of a successful Wall Street lawyer, and was polite and punctual. Haley describes the Muslims as having "manners and miens [that] reflected the Spartan personal discipline the organization demanded . . ."[32] While Malcolm hated the white man as the devil, he despised the "weak" black man who refused the effort to better himself: "The black man in the ghettoes . . . has to start self-correcting his own material, moral, and spiritual defects and evils. The black man needs to start his own program to get rid of drunkenness, drug addiction, prostitution. The black man in America has to lift up his own sense of values."[33]

This is dangerous talk. Liberals and psychiatrists need the weak-willed and the mentally sick so they have someone to care for, and something to do. If Malcolm had his way, all of these "helpers" would be unemployed, or worse. Here, then, is the basic conflict and contradiction between the Muslim and methadone; the former eliminates the problem, and thus the need for the white man and the doctor, by making the Negro self-responsible and self-reliant; the latter makes the white man and the doctor indispensable by making the Negro a permanent medical cripple and a lifelong patient, on the model laid down long ago by Benjamin Rush.

Malcolm, of course, understood and asserted—as indeed few black or white men could or would—that white men want the blacks to be on drugs, and that most black men who are on drugs want to be on them rather than off them. Freedom and self-determination are not only precious but arduous; most men, especially if not taught to value these things, want nothing to do with them. Malcolm X and Edmund Burke shared an appreciation of this important insight, this painful truth—that the state wants men to be weak and timid, not strong and proud.

This brings us face to face with the political dimension of the so-called drug problem, which Malcolm appraised in this way: "If some white man, or 'approved' black man, created a narcotic cure program as successful as the one conducted under the aegis of the Muslims, why, there would be government subsidy, and praise and spotlight, and headlines. But we were attacked instead."[34]

What Malcolm evidently failed to see, or see clearly enough, was that, by articulating and organizing his program as he did, he was, in fact, launching a religious war against greatly superior forces. I do not mean a religious war against Christianity. By rejecting Christianity and embracing Islam, the Muslims made their opposition to the "white man's religion" clear enough. But Christianity isn't the power it used to be, especially not in the United States. The religious war that Malcolm declared and waged, without quite realizing it, was the war against the religion of Medicine. After all, not only the whites, but most of his own black people, and all of the black leaders, believed—and continue to believe—that drug abuse is an illness. That is why they demand and demonstrate for "free" detoxification programs—and line up for methadone programs like Jews did for gas chambers. Malcolm saw this, but I am not sure he grasped the enormity of it all. Or perhaps he did and that is why, in the end, not long before he was killed, he rejected the Black Muslims, too, to whom, only a short while before, he gave all the credit for his resurrection from the living dead, and converted, once more, this time to Orthodox Islam. And he changed his name, too, this time to El Hajj Melik Shabazz—thus adopting, as his surname, the name of the legendary ancestors of the American Negroes from "Yacub's History."

The festering conflicts in Soviet society are between dissident individuals and groups—such as intellectuals, writers, and Jews—and the state; in our society, they are between dissident individuals and groups—such as the drug abusers, women, and blacks —and the state. In each case, the conflict is experienced by those who feel oppressed or persecuted by the state as moral or religious in character; and, in each case, the state tries to deny this experience and to redefine the conflict as political or preferably medical, and it often succeeds. The Russian government tries to narcotize its dissidents with alcohol, tobacco, work, and Communism; when these fail, it declares the deviants unpatriotic, enemies of the state, or mentally ill; and it deals with them accordingly, by incarcerating them in prisons or insane asylums. Similarly, the American government tries to narcotize its dissidents with alcohol, tobacco, work, money, and methadone; when these fail, it declares them incurably insane or permanently addicted; and it deals with them accordingly, by incarcerating some in prison, others in mental hospitals, and putting the rest on "methadone maintenance."

In short, heroin addiction, or any other illicit drug use, is no more "the problem" here than intellectual dissidence and the desire to emigrate are "the problem" in Russia. These "problems" are rather the pretexts for the latest assaults in the perennial wars that rulers wage against their subjects. Nor, perhaps, can they relent too far in pressing their advantage, lest the ruled—the people, the blacks, the whites, the addicts, the Jews wanting to leave Russia, all of us—were to forget their "proper place" and become "uppity." If only there had been a methadone maintenance program when Malcolm Little was a young man, Americans could have saved themselves incalculable troubles. How easy it would have been to seduce him into such a program!

Where does this leave our Presidents, our Governors, our National Institutes of Mental Health, our American Medical Association—and all the Negro leaders and organizations, too, save for the Black Muslims—all of whom push methadone?

It is ironic, but perhaps in the end hopeful, that—in the area of drug use and drug control (and in many other areas as well)—the Black Muslims, by reasserting the supremacy of internal controls over external, are actually defending individual self-determination against infantilizing state interference. In reasserting the traditional wisdom that "drug abuse" is simply bad manners—like being impolite, tardy, or unkempt—the Muslims find themselves in the company of such diverse groups as libertarians and conservatives,

patriots and Puritans, and also in competition with them. It remains to be seen how many black Americans want to compete
freely and fairly with their white fellow Americans, and vice versa;
and how many in each group prefer conquest or capitulation to
competition. In this balance may lie the future of our nation. Whatever the outcome, I believe it is now clear, and that it will be even
clearer in the future, that wherever else these parties may stand
on other matters, on drug abuse and drug addiction, the position of organized American medicine and of organized American
politics contradicts every principle and practice on which the
United States was founded; whereas that of the Black Muslims is
in the best American tradition.

8. FOOD ABUSE AND FOODAHOLISM: FROM SOUL WATCHING TO WEIGHT WATCHING

I have remarked earlier on man's basic moral scenario—the dramatic cycle of pollution and purification. Naturally, food and eating have a prominent role in this script: the most universal ceremonial of purification is fasting; and the most common ceremonial of self-indulgence or pollution is feasting. In general, the traditional religious response to, and method of coping with, grief or sorrow, is fasting; and with joy or happiness, it is feasting.

The importance of fasting in Christianity stems from the intensity of the imagery of humanity's essential sinfulness in this ideology; hence also the importance of fasting as a method of self-purification. The significance of these ideas and acts is reflected in our language. The entry for "fast" in the *Oxford English Dictionary* runs to eight and one-half columns, one of the longest for any word; the entry for "feast" is only two and one-half columns.

Moreover, this basic religious attitude toward fasting and feasting has been carried over, with appropriate linguistic and ceremonial changes but otherwise unchanged, into the modern medical attitude toward dieting. Indeed, the OED defines fasting as "Abstinence from food . . . as a religious observance," and dieting as a "prescribed course of food for medical or penal reasons." Thus, as medicine replaced religion (*as a religion*), dieting replaced fasting, and the treatment of obesity replaced the absolution for the sin of gluttony. All of this is, of course, but one facet of the pervasive medicalization of morals which has taken place during the past three centuries.

However obvious the parallels might seem between our former religious and our present medical positions concerning food, fasting, and feasting, they have escaped the notice of most modern scientists and physicians writing on this subject. For example, the preoccupation with the so-called problem of overweight, and the correspondingly much greater attention paid to weight reduction than to weight acquisition, are universally attributed to "scientific" considerations; in particular, to the higher incidence of "overnutrition" than "undernutrition" in the affluent societies and to the pathogenic effects of obesity. Furthermore, all authorities attribute the tendency to obesity, at least in part, to the deficiency of exercise in the modern life style. I do not dispute these interpretations as matters of fact. But I believe that every one of these "scientific explanations" conceals more than it explains.

The current medical emphasis on weight reduction parallels closely, as I have noted, the former religious emphasis on fasting. In the Middle Ages, food was, of course, not as plentiful or as easy to prepare as it is now; nor did people exercise so little. My point is that fasting then served, and that dieting now serves, the important ceremonial function of self-purification, but that this function is now concealed by the technical arguments in favor of weight reduction.

The purely medical perspective on nutrition cannot account for the greater preoccupation with slimness among women than among men. To explain this by invoking esthetic considerations is, of course, not to explain it at all; for the question remains why it should be so much more upsetting to women than to men to be a few pounds "overweight"? Is it because men treat women as "bodily"—that is to say, as sexual—objects? Each answer only pushes the question mark further down the page, without really answering it. I submit that concealed underneath all the nutritional, psychoanalytic, and male-chauvinist rhetoric lies the ancient presumption—the masculine fear and the feminine acceptance—of woman as an especially "polluted" person in need of special rites of "purification."

The notion of "feminine pollution" is an ancient belief.[1] The explanations and justifications for it have changed with the times, but the belief has not been dispelled. Indeed, in its present form it cannot be dispelled—because it is not acknowledged, either by women as individuals or by anthropologists and physicians as experts, that women's excessive preoccupation with being overweight and with dieting has anything at all to do with their being "unclean." I submit that the "overweight woman" is merely our contemporary version of the mythology of feminine pollution, some of whose earlier versions were menstruation, superior sexual powers, witchery, and "familiarity" with the devil—each with its appropriate purificatory precaution. We now look back at those earlier pollution-purification ceremonials and recognize them for what they were; but we stare, aphasic as it were, at our contemporary ceremonials—the massage parlors and weight-watching clubs, the diet manuals and health foods, the fraudulent physicians, "anorexics," and all the other medico-religious paraphernalia of the modern weight cult—and continue to treat the whole scene as if it posed a purely medical problem!

None of this is intended to deny any of the facts of physiology, or that certain medical principles and procedures might help some people to lose (or gain) weight. But it does not follow that, because medical techniques are used to regulate body weight, the regulation of body weight *is* a medical problem; any more than it follows that, because the electric chair may be used to execute criminals, the execution of criminals *is* a problem in electrical engineering.

Body weight lends itself perfectly to the contemporary passion for defining human qualities in terms of medical norms. The height-and-weight tables familiar to everyone today embody these standards. Significantly, however, although it is possible to deviate in four different directions from these norms, one of these deviations is stigmatized far more severely than are the other three. The person who is taller or shorter or lighter than the norm (unless so by a very wide margin), though "statistically abnormal," is accepted socially, largely because he or she is not defined as medically abnormal or sick. But woe to those who deviate in the fourth direction, that is, who are heavier than average: they are stigmatized socially as "overweight," esthetically as "repulsive," and medically as "sick." Indeed, society's, and especially the medical profession's, attitudes toward those who think the wrong thoughts (the insane), who take the wrong drugs (the addict), and who possess the wrong weight (the obese), display some remarkable similarities.

In the seventeenth century, a new medical specialty was created to study and control those who deviated from medical norms of social conduct; thus was psychiatry born. In the twentieth century, a new medical specialty was created to study and control those who deviated from medical norms of drug use; thus was drug-abuseology born. And in the 1960s, a new medical specialty was created to study and control those who deviated from medical norms of body weight; thus was bariatric medicine born. The professionalization of these exercises in malicious medical meddling into personal habits is important for several reasons: each of these pseudomedical enterprises redefines personal preference as a scientific and medical problem; conceals medical coercion as treatment; and, perhaps most importantly in the long run, creates an immense economic interest among physicians for fraudulently misrepresenting simple moral judgments as sophisticated medical diagnoses and crude coercions as refined therapeutic interventions.

For example, when psychiatry was young, its practitioners were at least correctly named "mad-doctors" and "keepers of madhouses"; but as these quacks gained power, their plain and informative names were replaced by the pompous professionalisms of "psychiatrist," "psychoanalysts," and "behavioral scientists." Similarly, physicians who counseled people to eat less or otherwise tried to help them reduce (or pretended to help them) were, until recently, called "fat doctors" and "pill pushers"; now there is a movement to rename them "bariatricians." In 1970, the American Society of Bariatric Physicians (from the Greek *baros* for weight) had a modest membership of 30; by 1972, the society's membership grew to an impressive 450.[2]

The first order of business for bariatricians is, of course, to manufacture "patients" suffering from the "disease" called "obesity." Wilmer A. Asher, M.D., Chairman of the Board of the American Society of Bariatric Physicians, evidently knows his business; and he thinks—like his "patients" eat—big. His initial estimate of the number of "patients" requiring his care and the care of his colleagues is staggering. "Somewhere between 30 and 60 million adult Americans," writes Asher, "are obese. If the same number of our citizens were afflicted with measles or smallpox, it would be considered an epidemic."[3]

Asher has not simply made up these figures; they have been

made up for him by other physicians and nutritionists who have been trying, with considerable success, to persuade the American people that obesity is our most common illness. The following sentence from the foreword to a prestigious symposium on obesity, held at the University of California Medical Center in San Francisco in 1967, is typical: "Certainly, in the United States obesity is the gravest sign of malnutrition when it is realized that 25 to 36 percent of the adult population in the United States is 10 percent or more overweight."[4]

In a postscript to this symposium, entitled "Obesity: A Gross National Product,"[5] while much of the blame for this "disease" is placed at the door of America's decadent affluence, we are at least also reminded of the financial stakes that physicians and the drug and food industries have in this sort of medical racketeering. Among the more interesting figures are these: the food industry spends more than $1 billion a year on advertising; at the same time, the sales of low-calorie diet foods are increasing rapidly, with the sales of Metracal (a special food supplement that has since sunk into oblivion) rising to $150 million within two years of its introduction; vitamin sales total about $200 million per year, and the sale of drugs that allegedly suppress the appetite come to about $80 million. In relation to the latter item, it is worth noting that while the amphetamines have now entered into the Valhalla of "Dangerous Drugs" whose illicit possession in New York State can now earn one a permanent prison diet, the medical use of these and related drugs continues to be a big business. Thus, the 1973 edition of the *Physicians' Desk Reference,* the standard guide to all American pharmaceutical preparations, lists, in its "Drug Classification Index," no fewer than thirty-four different preparations classified as "Anorexics"; these drugs are also cross-indexed as "Anti-Obesity Preparations."[6]

The foregoing brief review of the present state of the art of obesity management suggests that there may be a greater future in bariatric than in psychiatric medicine: bariatricians will easily be able to claim everyone as their patients; and the possibilities for the involuntary diagnosis and treatment of weight problems is enough to boggle the imagination. For, obviously, to a conscientious bariatrician anyone *heavier* than a Gandhi would be a "case of obesity," actual, latent, or potential; and anyone *like* a Gandhi would be a "case of nervous anorexia" or "psychogenic food refusal," and hence also a proper subject for medical treatment. Whatever deviance the psychiatrization of American society might fail to detect, the bariatrization of it will surely pick up and correct.

Like other medical scapegoats, and especially like involuntary mental patients who do not want to be patients at all, the "obese" also often reject—if not in word then in deed—the patient role. Their actions communicate a desire to be or remain fat or, perhaps more accurately, to weigh more than others think they should. Although pleading for more authority to practice fat-doctoring, and perhaps to exclude others from this practice, Asher himself characterizes his potential patients in these revealing words: "Obese patients are difficult. They don't stay on diets; they lie to their doctors; they don't keep appointments. If their physicians are too hard on them, they go to another doctor. If they are too easy on them, they stay fat. Often the physician fails to help the fat patient."[7] Asher thus almost says, but does not quite say, two things: first, that in view of their uncooperative attitude, obese patients—like madmen and addicts—would be best treated involuntarily in closed institutions; and second, that although the physician *often* fails to help his obese patients, he *never* fails to help himself—to the patient's (or insurance company's, or some other third party's) money.

As in psychiatry, here also we encounter the physician labeling the patient a "liar"—when in fact it is the physician himself (and his organization and profession) who is engaged in the most massive mendacity. For it is the physician who calls people who eat intemperately—if that is why they are fat—"sick"; who calls people who do not want to see him—as revealed by their "missing" appointments—"patients"; and who calls advising people to eat less —by giving them "diets"—a form of "medical treatment."

Certain parallels between obesity and addiction are, of course, quite obvious, and are often acknowledged—sometimes even emphasized—by laymen and professionals alike. Overweight persons

are called "carboholics" and "foodaholics"; many declare themselves as helpless vis-à-vis food as alcoholics are vis-à-vis alcohol,
and seek relief from submitting themselves to authorities whose
coercions they shamelessly seek and invite. Natalie Allon—who,
incidentally, is one of the few persons writing on obesity to have
clearly rejected the fraudulent medicalization of this problem—
notes that "weight-losing groups offer an attractive alternative healing system for the 'disease' or 'sin' of overweight. Many dieters
find comfort in submission to the external authority of the group."[8]
The similarities between Weight Watchers (and other such
groups) and Alcoholics Anonymous is obvious—except that the
foodaholic cannot abstain completely from food; however—and
this is more to the point—the foodaholic can adopt the substitute habit ("addiction") of dieting, just as the alcoholic can
adopt the substitute habit ("addiction") of abstaining. Allon
quotes a Trim-Downer who describes herself in this way: "I guess
I am just hooked on dieting for life and I am always looking for
the magical cure—the final end to my dieting mania when I will be
thin forever."[9]

Besides the medical experts, most weight reducers—like most
alcohol rehabilitators and most drug-abuseologists—are themselves
ex-addicts. Their qualification lies in their having been "sinners"
who have become "saints." This mythicoreligious process of "purification" by overcoming "pollution"—which I described earlier[10]
—is enacted in dieting perhaps even more clearly and dramatically
than it is in abstaining from alcohol or other drugs. Allon's account
of it is as instructive as it is accurate: "The morally good Trim-
Downer is one who attempts to perfect a better and better body.
To be such a supreme good, the final cure of a thin body must
evolve from a fat body. The holiness is in the act of cleansing. To
be a saint, one must start as a sinner."[11]

Consistent with this model, the saved sinners try to save others,
and as many as possible. "Trim-Down healers were self-styled experts whose basic qualification to lead weight-losing groups was
the fact that they had been healed from their own fatness by the
Trim-Down diet plan. . . . Besides a [basic] diet, the quasi-

religious service of group dieting was the primary method of operation of the Trim-Down healing system."[12]

The appearance and acceptance on the modern medical scene of a class of allegedly or ostensibly "scientific" experts whose authority depends solely on their having been "medical sinners"—that is, on having been alcoholics, drug addicts, or foodaholics—has not received the attention it deserves, except, perhaps, in humor. I have heard my colleagues remark banteringly, more than once, that they no longer advise their sons to become doctors or lawyers; they suggest, instead, that they become "ex-addicts."

The real import and impact of the ex-alcoholic, ex-addict, and ex-foodaholic as paramedical expert lies in this: each symbolizes the medical profession's abdication from genuine scientific and technical standard setting and performance judging; it encourages physicians, despite the remarkable recent scientific achievements of their profession, to reject their reliance on evidence and inference, technology and truth, and to substitute for them the pomp and glory of a fake religion; and, finally, it propels medicine ever more deeply into the arms of the state, where, from its crushing embrace, it first becomes imbecilic from cerebral anoxia and then mercifully suffocates.

I have argued that the contemporary mania about drug abuse and the associated persecution of drug abusers is a modern version of what Charles Mackay called "extraordinary popular delusions and crowd madnesses."[13] If this view is valid, we should expect to find certain parallels, in addition to those already noted, between the persecution of drug abusers on the one hand and the persecution of witches and Jews on the other; in particular, we should find the imposition of a scapegoated identity spreading from an initially discrete group—such as helpless women, poor Jews, or black heroin addicts—to other groups, for example, Christian schismatics, non-Aryans of all kinds, or young persons with long hair.

Once it becomes accepted that a particular group of persons—for example, witches or Jews—is "dangerous," the crusade to eliminate each and every one of its members tends to generate victims from other groups as well. Every major wave of scapegoating has exhibited this characteristic—which is no doubt a consequence of the unleashing of the base human passions of envy, greed, revenge, and plain murderousness. What started as the persecution of a few witches and heretics became, in the hands of the inquisitors, far-reaching campaigns against dissident Christians of all kinds, Jews and Mohammedans, the poor and the rich—against anyone who provoked another's anger or envy.

In the American war against drugs there have already been two clearly discernible periods during which the identity of the scapegoated drug was first displaced from one to another and then spread from one to several others. The first of these is perhaps a special case, but is relevant nevertheless. I refer to the transformation of the war against alcohol, after the repeal of Prohibition, into the war, first against marijuana, and then against other "dangerous drugs." The second identity diffusion of the scapegoat began around 1960, since which time we have witnessed the war against drugs fan out from marijuana and LSD to heroin, cocaine, barbiturates, and amphetamines.

The escalation of this "war against harmful substances" has finally reached the point where the "enemy" is food itself! The martial metaphor is not mine, as the following example shows.

On October 6, 1971, the Associated Press reported a news dispatch headlined: "Fish and Chips the Enemy in USAF's 'Battle of the Bulge.'" The martial metaphor here leans partly on the fact that one of the combatants in this engagement is the United States Air Force. The identity of the other combatant, of the *enemy*—not placed between quotation marks in the report, and hence presumably a literal rather than a metaphorical enemy—is food; indeed, foreign food, as we learn even before reading the report, which, with some omissions, I reproduce below.

> The U. S. Air Force is fighting the battle of the bulging waistline among its ground crews in Britain. One target is fish and chips. Chunks of fried cod nestling in French fries are banned at two of the six big U.S. bases, Lakenheath and Mildenhall. Nearby fish and chip shops there have been put off limits. Similar action may be taken elsewhere. "The trouble is that many personnel fresh from the States find fish and chips quite appetizing," one sergeant explained.

. . . All airmen at South Ruislip Base outside London are being weighed to see how much damage English food has done. The fatties will get orders warning them against the dishes. "Hundreds of airmen throughout Britain are going to be found overweight," a spokesman said. Except for those with medical problems, fatties who disobey orders and still give in to the lure of fish and chips will be confined to Air Force hospitals until they kick the habit.[14]

One hardly knows where to begin "analyzing" this passage, which compares favorably with some of George Orwell's most imaginative scenes out of *1984* or *Animal Farm.* Let me begin by noting that, even after the same story was printed, in somewhat shorter form, in *Parade*[15] (which is said to be read by some 25 million Americans), I do not recall seeing a single complaint or protest against this incredible infringement of the civil liberties not only of the alleged American "fatties" but also of the British shopkeepers whose establishments were boycotted by an order of the U. S. Air Force. Indeed, not only was there no objection to this story, but it was presented, especially in *Parade,* in a manner that clearly conveyed the magazine's support for what must have appeared to most people as an "obviously" reasonable and well-intentioned policy: "To help their men win the battle of the bulge, authorities . . . declared the local fish and chips shops off-limits," is the way *Parade* had put it.

While this sort of helpfulness may be obvious to those who approve of this sort of medical meddling, it is not so at all to those who don't. And since I don't, I find a wealth of interesting information in both the content and the language of this story.

First, American citizens are deprived here of ingesting a substance that is not a drug but a food; nevertheless, they are deprived of it on grounds that are indistinguishable from those used to justify the prohibition of so-called dangerous drugs.

Second, the prohibited food is a foreign food—indeed, one of the national dishes of the friendly foreign country in which the airmen are stationed. The argument that fish and chips is banned because of its high fat content is, of course, quite unconvincing. Hot dogs, apple pie, and ice cream are not mentioned in the news dispatches, and presumably continued to be available to the airmen at their own bases. The Associated Press report actually refers explicitly to the "damage English food has done" to the airmen. English food, not American. The parallel here with the promotion of tobacco because it is American and the prohibition of marijuana because it is foreign is a close one: Hot dogs should be "legalized" because they are part of our cultural heritage; fish and chips should be declared "dangerous" and prohibited (and perhaps made available by physician's prescription as treatment for the disease of Anglophobia) because they are un-American.

Third, the language used to describe this food is strikingly similar to the language used to describe "dangerous" drugs. The fish "nestles" in French fries; it does "damage" to the airmen, who give in to its "lure"; the scapegoated persons are called "fatties," who are prohibited from eating fish and chips, and are imprisoned in Air Force hospitals until "they kick the habit"!

Fourth, no one seems to have considered the moral, legal, and civil rights aspects of this situation, as regards both the American airmen and the British merchants. The airmen are handled just as dangerous madmen or addicts are—by incarceration in hospitals. The merchants are attacked just as enemies are in peacetime—by a boycott against their products. Yet, as far as I know, there has been no protest against this insult to British eating habits and infringement of British rights.

Furthermore, putting fish and chips shops off-limits for American servicemen in England, but not putting Kentucky Fried Chicken shops—or the Lums chain, which also serves fish and chips—off-limits for them in America, has certainly done nothing *for* the weight control of American servicemen; what it has done *to* their sense of equity and fair play, freedom and dignity—in short, to their appreciation of all the values for whose defense they are supposedly in uniform—one can only conjecture.

Fifth, and last, I want to protest against the utter debasement—the politicization, psychiatrization, and penologization—of medicine and medical institutions implicit in the procedures here described. Eating British as against American food is treated here as if it were a medical problem, and as if overeating (not otherwise defined) were an especially serious medical problem, requiring "hospitalization." Moreover, in a quite bizarre conclusion of the story, we are informed that airmen who "give in to the lure of fish and chips . . . *except for those with medical problems* . . . will be confined to Air Force hospitals . . ." (emphasis added). This policy, if true, condemns all those responsible for it as mendacious medical criminals. In traditional American institutional psychiatry, and in modern Soviet mental health practices, the medical prostitutes of the system at least *pretend* that their victims are sick, and that they are confined *because* they are sick. Here, however, it is emphasized that those genuinely ill will be excluded from hospital care (which presumably they do not need, outpatient treatment being more appropriate for them), "hospitalization" being reserved for those who are *without* medical problems.

Truly, the "plague" of drug abuse and drug addiction threatens America and Americans. But, as this spread of the medical persecution from masturbation to marijuana and thence to fish and chips shows, the danger in this plague lies not in the disease, which is nonexistent, but in the cure, which is unrestrained medical barbarism disguised and defined as diagnosis, prevention, protection, hospitalization, and treatment.

To appreciate how very logically the "criminalization" of fish and chips follows from the totalitarian medical perspective on drug abuse, obesity, and all human problems, I want to turn next from the "hospital treatment" of "addiction to fish and chips" to the surgical treatment of obesity regardless of the national origin of the food that "causes" it.

The medical perspective on habits logically locates the nature of the "problem"—whether it be self-abuse or food abuse—in the "affected" organ rather than in the person who has the habit. It is very much as if a person who speaks English with a foreign accent because he has lived abroad as a child were subjected to some sort of "reconstructive surgery" on his mouth, tongue, and teeth, to correct his faulty speech habits. The manifest absurdity of this sort of surgery, and the even more manifest sadism of the surgeons who perform it and the gullibility of the patients who submit to it, have not dampened the recurring enthusiasm for ever-new surgical "cures" of this kind. Thus, in the nineteenth century, clitoridectomy in girls and circumcision in boys were accepted methods of treatment for masturbation. Amputation of the penis was advocated, as recently as 1891, by one of the presidents of the (British) Royal College of Surgeons.[16] In the twentieth century surgeons continue—for certain "bad habits" of thought, speech, and conduct called "schizophrenia"—to mutilate a perfectly healthy organ, the brain. The discoverer of this "treatment," Egas Moniz, received the Nobel Prize for it. The treatment itself, called lobotomy or leucotomy, has also been used on addicts.

And so we come to the surgical treatment of obesity—the "bad habit" of eating too much. Since without a properly functioning digestive tract one cannot become obese, medical science locates the "lesion" of the disease called "obesity" in the digestive tract, and goes to work on "correcting" it. Incredible? Not at all. If physicians, patients, and politicians all agree that overeating is a medical problem, who is left to stop them from acting on their sincerely held belief? Indeed, why should anyone stop them? Married people are often said to "deserve each other"; perhaps so do patients and their doctors. Moreover, as there are many more patients than physicians, if the patients are victimized, they must play an important part in their own victimization—a victimization which, we know only too well, is often the consequence of their trying to evade their responsibilities for self-critical thinking and self-disciplined living.

The surgical treatment of obesity was developed by two Los Angeles surgeons, J. Howard Payne and Loren T. DeWind, who began to use so-called intestinal bypass operations in 1956. Their first procedure was a jejunocolic shunt, connecting the jejunum to the colon, thus "bypassing" and rendering non-functional a large portion of the small intestine and some portion of the large intestine. However, by 1969, because of its adverse effects, they discontinued this procedure and replaced it with a less extensive bypass, the jejunoileal shunt. Operations for obesity have since enjoyed a considerable vogue both in the United States and in Canada. My aim in what follows is, of course, not so much to review this literature as to ridicule and criticize it. I will, however, cite some of the statements of the most respected authorities in this field, in order both to present their views and to illustrate the physicians' seemingly irresistible impulses to control their patients.

In the August 1969 issue of the *American Journal of Surgery,* Payne and DeWind summarize their fifteen-year experience in the field: "1. A jejunoileal shunt is of distinct benefit in selected patients for whom the obese state has become a hazard to health. 2. It is not the procedure one does because an obese patient is 25 to 50 pounds overweight. 3. Inasmuch as a high degree of cooperation is essential, a relationship of mutual respect, trust, and responsibility must be present between the physician and patient. A hostile attitude on the part of the patient cannot be tolerated. . . ."[17]

A "hostile attitude" on the part of the physician evidently *can* be tolerated. Yet Payne and DeWind preach the virtue of "cooperation" and "mutual respect" between patient and doctor.

In the formal discussion printed following the Payne-DeWind paper, Jack M. Farris, M.D., another Los Angeles surgeon, offers these comments: "Five years ago, when this same subject was being discussed, I suggested that perhaps the same goal could be achieved by simply wiring people's teeth together, as if they had a fractured jaw. I must retract this approach, however, because I have now discovered that to eliminate 100 pounds of excess fat, the energy content of which is about 400,000 calories, takes from six months to one year of complete fasting. Consequently, the man Dr. Payne discussed, who lost 380 pounds, would have had to have his teeth wired together for approximately four years to achieve the same result."[18]

Said in jest but meant in earnest: wiring people's teeth together to make them lose weight! But, then, physicians used to strap spiked chastity belts on boys' genitals to make them stop masturbating; and still chop off people's frontal lobes to make them stop uttering disturbing thoughts.

In general, one's judgment about the moral aspects of these procedures—beginning with what one defines as a "problem" and what criteria one selects for determining what is and is not morally permissible as a "solution"—will depend on one's rank-ordering of values, especially with respect to such notions as health, individual liberty, and medical coercion. I personally abhor all the interventions I have been discussing. But in my mind the crucial criterion for judging the morality of such interventions is not whether I adore or abhor them, but whether they are performed on fully informed consenting clients or not. (Children are, by definition, nonconsenting clients; because they are deprived of the legal right to contract, they are "involuntary patients.") I thus believe—and I believe that anyone valuing personal autonomy cannot with consistency hold otherwise—that individuals should be left free to decide whether they want to define themselves as "patients" because they masturbate, have thoughts that scare them, or overeat, and should be left free to decide whether they want to submit themselves to physicians for mutilating their bodies in an effort to "purify" them of their "pollutions." Freedom of religion should thus include not only theological religion but also medical, surgical, and psychiatric religion. Since I view "involuntary treatment" as analogous to involuntary religious conversion, I need hardly say anything more about my objections to it—regardless of the medical benefits attributed to it by its proponents.

Dr. Farris' foregoing remarks deserve one more comment. His calling attention to the immense caloric reservoir represented by 100 pounds of body fat dramatizes, if not the "wages of sin," then at least the consequences of long-ingrained habits. To become overweight by hundreds of pounds obviously requires long years of practice in overeating; hence, we should compare obesity, not to a disease like diabetes, but to a hard-won skill, like playing the violin expertly. Clearly, it would be impossible to "cure" a violin virtuoso of his "compulsive" violin playing by trying to prevail on him to stop, especially so long as he did not "really" want to stop. But let us assume that, despite some such state of affairs, he becomes convinced, because of intense social pressure on him, that he ought to stop playing. He might then be a willing candidate for the surgical treatment of compulsive violin playing—which might consist of the amputation of some or all fingers of one or both hands. A considerable surgical literature could then develop, different surgeons advocating the amputation of fewer or more fingers, and of more or less of any one finger. Clearly, we have barely scratched the surface of a surgical lode rich in the possibilities of the treatment of habits by means of "reconstructive" operations.

To be sure, these "cures" cost something, even if Blue Cross pays for them. "It is amazing to me," comments Dr. Farris—whose remark about wiring teeth together must hide a heart of gold—"that although the jejunocolic fistula has really no place in the treatment of obesity . . . since it is incompatible with health and vigor, it is still being used in a great number of centers."[19] It is not amazing to me. But I agree that perhaps medical schools should teach the anatomy of Pandora's Box no less intensively than they teach the anatomy of other containers with whose contents they expect the educated physician to be familiar.

The surgical treatment of obesity by intestinal bypass operations has now been practiced for nearly twenty years. Its present professional status may be inferred from the following comment by Harry H. LeVeen, M.D., on a paper on the jejunoileal bypass published in the *American Journal of Surgery* in 1972: "Surgical therapy for morbid obesity is attractive because medical therapy almost always fails. If these patients are compulsive eaters, so-called food alcoholics, they eat for relief of anxiety. Obviously, diets which disallow foods are anxiety producing. Surgery becomes the more acceptable therapy from a psychological viewpoint."[20]

The image of a fat person as nothing but an adipose body containing irresistible impulses for gorging itself with food is here neither articulated nor debated; it is simply taken for granted. It is perhaps also taken for granted by "the American public," insofar at least as that public's sentiments may be inferred from the way things are presented in *Time* magazine. In April 1972, *Time* printed a long story on the surgical treatment of obesity from which the reader could have easily gathered the impression that the only thing wrong with the operation is that it is sometimes "abused" by unscrupulous surgeons. Some, we learn, even fail to make the proper anastomoses, or surgical reconnections, between the severed ends of the patient's intestinal tract, with fatal results, of course. Here is the way *Time* explains how this operation works: "[The] shortening of the digestive tract cuts down on caloric absorption, enabling excessively overweight people to shed pounds regardless of how much they eat. To perform it, the surgeon severs the small intestine near the end of the jejunum and connects it to the ileum just above the beginning of the colon. This in turn reduces the length of the active small intestine from 23 feet to a mere 30 inches, drastically lessening the time it takes for food to pass through the system. This reduces the amount of digested material that can be absorbed through the intestinal walls."[21]

This sounds very nice and scientific. Calories don't count. Willpower doesn't count. And medical insurance no doubt pays for it. It is much more refined, too, than the disgusting Roman "treatment" for overeating: namely, tickling the back of the throat with a feather to induce vomiting. We are past such filthy habits.

In any case, tickling one's throat to induce vomiting is too much like tickling one's genitals to induce orgasm. These are things a person does for himself and by himself, and must, therefore, be condemned—and prohibited, if possible. We must, after all, never be alone and never be self-controlled (however peculiarly so). The heteronomous ethic demands that someone else control us: a sexual partner our orgasms; a surgeon our obesity. Thus we have the bypass operation for overeating—a kind of once-and-for-all abortion of the intestinal contents; a circumcision of the small intestine; a lobotomy of the digestive tract. All this is legal and therapeutic. The physicians who perform these operations are famous and respected surgeons, who publish their researches in the most prestigious medical journals. At the same time, ordinary people who sell amphetamines are heading for life imprisonment. Such is life in the Age of Madness, where the ruling religion is Scientific Medicine.

III. Pharmacracy: Medicine as Social Control

9. MISSIONARY MEDICINE: HOLY WARS ON UNHOLY DRUGS

The point of view on medicine which I have been developing, here and elsewhere,[1] requires a radical revision of our traditional sentimental image of this profession as one simply devoted to healing the sick. It requires, in particular, that we supplement it with the image of a profession that, though primarily medical and hence concerned with healing the sick, is also religious and magical and hence concerned with rituals of pollution and purification; and is also political and penological, and hence concerned with the social control of personal conduct.

The activities of the Nazi physicians, for which many were hanged at Nuremberg, were, unfortunately, not the aberrations of a holy healing profession imposed upon it by the terrors of a totalitarian regime, but, on the contrary, were the characteristic, albeit exaggerated, expressions of the medical profession's traditional functions as instruments of social control. Physicians had assisted the Inquisition; supported the military efforts of all nations; and regularly serve, in all modern countries, as an extralegal police force to control deviance—especially through involuntary psychiatric interventions. The medical profession's war against certain drugs—and in support of others—is then just one more episode (at present perhaps one of the most important ones) in its long history of participation in religious, national, and political conflicts. Instead of reviewing the history of this struggle, which I have covered elsewhere, I shall only mention a few typical battles between the forces of missionary medicine and its enemies.

A typical, relatively early, example of the prostitution of the medical role in the interests of repressing certain "deviants" by attacking their drug-taking habits is an article published in 1921 in the *Journal of the American Medical Association*. Its author, Thomas S. Blair—a physician and the chief of the Bureau of Drug Control of the Pennsylvania Department of Health—gave his essay the wonderfully revealing title "Habit Indulgence in Certain Cactaceous Plants among the Indians."[2] The Indians, of course, had

no *Journal of the Indian Peyote Association* in which they could
have published an article on "Habit Indulgence in the Fermented
Juice of Certain Grapes among the Americans." Right from the
start, then, the Indians were peyote addicts—while the Americans
laughed all the way to the speakeasies. And so it has been ever
since, except that today, whites, blacks, and Puerto Ricans—that
is, all of us—are treated like the Indians were fifty years ago; and
the only ones laughing all the way to the hospitals and halls of
legislatures are the physicians and politicians.

Beginning with its crucially defamatory title—in which language
is used early and decisively to debase another religion as a superstition and its most important ceremony as a "habit indulgence"—
Blair's entire article is full of the sorts of mendacities that have
always characterized missionary medical writings, especially with
respect to subjects such as masturbation, mental illness, and drug
abuse.

Actually, the use of peyote was basic to the pre-Columbian
religious practices of Aztec and other Mexican Indians. Both
the Spanish civil authorities and the Spanish Inquisition tried to
abolish its use, and both were unsuccessful. Edward M. Brecher
summarizes the vast literature on peyotism as follows: "Anthropologists are quite generally agreed that the migration of peyote and
its associated religion northward to the beleaguered Indians of
the United States brought many advantages. The peyote cult required total abstinence from alcohol—and there is abundant evidence that Indians who accepted peyotism did in fact abandon
alcohol in substantial numbers." In addition, since peyote was
shared by many Indian tribes, it was "a step toward pan-Indianism,
the awareness of common interests that is a dominant theme of
American Indian culture today."[3]

Those reading only the medical literature on peyote would, however, not suspect any of this. The American Medical Association
—the Vatican of the American Medical Church—had picked up the
torch dropped by the Spanish Inquisition and has never relinquished its hostility toward non-alcoholic pharmacomythologies.
In the article cited above, Blair asserts—as if it constituted an ir-
refutable argument—that the "government has investigated the

use of peyote and found its evil effects to parallel the Oriental abuse of cannabis. The addict becomes indolent, immoral, and worthless."⁴ We should recall that Blair wrote this article, and the *Journal of the American Medical Association* published it, while the American people, under Prohibition, drank more liquor than ever before; and while the American medical profession participated in the liquor business by selling drink through prescriptions. This situation, continuing to our day—and becoming increasingly more international in scope—is similar to the situation of pre-Reformation Christianity, the priests preaching abstinence and continence, while selling indulgences and otherwise indulging themselves in the vices on whose prohibitions they battened.

The themes of religious warfare and of missionary medicine— that is, of Christianity against the native Indian church, of alcoholism against peyotism—often buried under the fake medical facts and scientific explanations of the drug experts, emerge here with hardly any disguise at all, as in a dream. "Missionary workers in the Southwest," Blair writes, "are becoming seriously concerned over the spreading use of mescal buttons, whether called peyote or by other name."⁵ Lest the reader be left in some doubt about what business this is of the missionaries, Blair explains that "certain Sons of Belial, taking advantage of the tendency of the Indian to religious ceremonial, have been industriously spreading the word among the tribes that partaking of the peyote enables the addict [sic] to communicate with the Great Spirit. It is true that certain Mexican tribes have long had a superstitious reverence for mescal buttons and have used them on occasion in religious ceremonials; and this old superstition gave the commercial dope vendor a great opportunity among the Indians in the United States. This has been carried so far that the 'Peyote Church' has actually been incorporated, the members being devotees, who gather for an orgy of frenzy, far worse than the cocaine parties held among the negroes."⁶

As recently as in 1921, an American physician could write that it was not the American government that had "exploited" the Indians, but those who sold them the peyote they used in their religious ceremonials! Actually, it was the "land speculators, who coveted the tribal lands where the peyote rites were practiced, and Christian missionaries [who] sought to have peyote outlawed. They scored modest successes in a few state legislatures. They were less successful, however, in getting anti-peyote legislation through Congress; anthropologists and friends of the Indians joined with the Indians themselves to defeat such legislation year after year."[7]

Among these friends of the Indians, physicians and medical organizations were conspicuous by their absence; and they continue to be conspicuous by their absence from among those whose voices oppose, rather than support, the holy medical wars on the "plague" of drug abuse.

Blair's rhetoric offers a typical example and a characteristic precursor of what was to follow during the next half-century. In indicting peyote, the Indians who use it, and the "dope vendors" who provide it, Blair—and the American Medical Association, whose views he was obviously articulating—indicts himself and his profession for intolerance of drug habits differing from those of the majority. This intolerance has continued to characterize organized American medicine. Blair complains of "the great difficulty in suppressing this habit," never for a minute doubting the moral legitimacy of the efforts to suppress it! Has the American Medical Association ever doubted the wisdom or legitimacy of the efforts to suppress the use of marijuana or opiates? Pharmacological prohibitionists, like all religious proselytizers, are singularly free of the self-restraints that characterize the behavior of those who can entertain doubts about the legitimacy of their own coercive tactics. "*There is no doubt* [emphasis added]," Blair concludes, "that the Gandy bill or similar legislation [to criminalize the use of peyote] is needed for the protection not only of the Indian, but of the whites as well."[8]

The American Medical Association's position on self-medication and drug controls has at least been consistent during the past fifty years. It has never told the truth about drugs (as that "truth" was seen and recorded by contemporary chemists and pharmacologists), if telling it was in conflict with government policies or with the Association's desire to gain exclusive control over the use of certain substances. For example, when in 1944 the New York Academy of Medicine issued its report on marijuana which declared its use "completely harmless," the *Journal of the American Medical Association* "hurled a few invectives at the Academy, warning that 'Public officials will do well to disregard this unscientific study and to continue to regard marijuana as a menace wherever it is purveyed.' "[9]

As I write this, the nation's highest-ranking official drug-abuseologist is Dr. Jerome H. Jaffe, President Nixon's "drug czar." Between 1966 and 1971, Jaffe was the psychiatrist employed by the state of Illinois to administer that state's "drug program"; that is, he persecuted "addicts" on behalf of the Illinois state government.[10] In 1971, he was appointed by President Nixon to head a new Special Action Office of Drug Abuse Prevention; that is, he became the Grand Inquisitor of the national anti-drug crusade. Hence, his assertions can be credited with scant factual validity, but must be seen instead as serving the purpose of "reaffirming the faith"—in this case, the faith in the drug ceremonials of contemporary American society.

My reason for this judgment has, of course, nothing to do with Dr. Jaffe's "medical competence." It has to do instead with the much more basic and simple fact that Jaffe does not himself define what constitutes drug abuse, but accepts the definition of this "condition" provided for him—and for all of us—by American politicians and voters; and, having accepted that definition, lends his knowledge and skill to implementing the policies implicit in it.

By now, this is, of course, a time-honored psychiatric role and scenario: that is, the prominent psychiatrist as legitimizer and executioner of the American politician's will. Only a few years ago, and in a closely related context, having to do with sex rather than with drugs, Manfred Guttmacher—one of the most prominent psychiatrists in America at the time and the recipient of the American Psychiatric Association's coveted Isaac Ray Award—asserted: "If it is considered the will of the majority that large numbers of sex offenders . . . be indefinitely deprived of their liberty and supported at the expense of the state, I readily yield to that judgment."[11]

Jaffe has, as far as I know, not said anything like this. But actions speak louder than words: through his actions, he has come down squarely in favor of the identical judgment and policy with respect to "drug offenders." His very ·"office" supplies a professional justification for politically mandated anti-drug policies and is thus one of the instruments for depriving "drug abusers" of their liberty and supporting them indefinitely at the expense of the state!

How missionary medicine corrupts scientific medicine—with Jaffe playing the role of missionary—is strikingly illustrated by the changing portrayals of opium and morphine in the most widely accepted and used textbook of pharmacology in the English language—*The Pharmacological Basis of Therapeutics,* by Louis Goodman and Alfred Gilman.

In the first edition, published in 1941, the pharmacology of opiates is presented by the authors in a chapter entitled "Morphine and Other Opium Alkaloids," the first paragraph of which reads as follows:

> In 1680 Sydenham wrote, "Among the remedies which it has pleased Almighty God to give man to relieve his sufferings, none is so universal and so efficacious as opium." This appraisal is still true today. If it were necessary to restrict the choice of drugs to a very few, the great majority of physicians would place the opium alkaloids, particularly morphine, at the head of the list. Morphine is unequalled as an analgesic and its indispensable uses in medicine and surgery are well defined.[12]

A brief discussion of opiate addiction and its treatment is included in this chapter; but there is no special chapter on drug addiction and the term "drug abuse" is nowhere in sight.

The second edition, still written solely by the same authors, was published in 1955. There is no significant change in the presentation of the pharmacology of opiates and the paragraph quoted above is reprinted unchanged.[13]

The third edition, published in 1965, is edited by Goodman and Gilman, the various chapters being written by different authors. The chapter on opiates, now titled "Narcotic Analgesics," is written by Jerome H. Jaffe, a psychiatrist—a remarkable choice in view of the previous identification of morphine as having "indispensable uses in medicine and surgery." Obviously, morphine is not a drug used *in* psychiatry, in the sense in which it is used in medicine and surgery. On the contrary, psychiatry is identified with attempts to make people *not* use opiates. Indeed, there is a new chapter in this edition on "Drug Addiction and Drug Abuse," not surprisingly also written by Jaffe. Is this not like a Nazi writing about Jews, or a Jew writing about the Nazis? But, then, when the Nazis were in power, who else but a Nazi could write about the Jews in Germany? And since the Nazis have been defeated, who else but their enemy can be an accredited expert on them? Or, to draw another analogy, Jaffe contributing a chapter to a textbook of therapeutics on how to use opium is like me contributing a chapter to a textbook of psychiatry on how to use electroshock or commitment. And yet neither Goodman nor Gilman, nor perhaps anyone else, has felt that there was anything wrong with one of the nation's leading opponents of opiates writing on their use. This is how far psychiatry and the war on drugcraft have contaminated the contemporary writing of pharmacology.

Although the pharmacology of opium did not change between 1955 and 1970, and no superior analgesics were developed during that period, Jaffe has twice changed the paragraph quoted above. In the third edition, he cites Sydenham, and then adds: "This appraisal needs only slight modification today."[14] In the fourth edition, published in 1970, he still cites Sydenham, but the approving comment about opium, toned down from the second to the third edition, is deleted.[15] And in both the third and fourth editions, the two sentences extolling morphine are replaced by a fresh text about "newer agents" of analgesia, further downgrading the opiates. As the political totalitarians have shown us how to bring history up to date, so the therapeutic totalitarians show us how to bring pharmacology up to date.

Of course, the same considerations which I have cited with respect to Jaffe apply to all of our officially accredited experts on drug abuse: they are the high priests of the crusade against illegal, psychoactive drugs—just as, say, Timothy Leary was the high priest of the crusade for them. In short, I maintain that our so-called drug experts are in effect merchants of politically mandated medical mendacities regarding substances feared and rejected by our society.

There is, of course, a vigorous public demand for such merchants, and a corresponding demand for silencing those who want to sell or tell the truth. In February 1970 an editorial in the *Syracuse Post-Standard* not only heaped lavish praise on Governor Rockefeller's "$265-million crash program to fight drug addiction," but also urged "one man in total charge of the program armed with almost dictatorial powers . . . a czar, if you will." The editorial concluded with this revealing warning: "One of the very first things that needs to be done is to rid the State University and the public schools of every faculty member or employee who publicly, or privately, defends the right of students to use any kinds of drugs. . . ."[16] Not even aspirin?

As clerical missionaries produced pagans out of natives, the better to be able to convert them to faithful Christians, so the clinical missionaries produce drug abusers out of persons with deviant drug habits, the better to be able to convert them to normal alcohol drinkers and tobacco smokers. Here is a current example—again chosen almost at random from the daily press—to illustrate how drug-abuseologists manufacture "drug freaks" and some of their astounding experiences.

Early in January 1968, Raymond P. Shafer, then the Governor of Pennsylvania and subsequently chairman of President Nixon's Marijuana Commission, announced that six college students stared at the sun while under the influence of LSD and were blinded as a result. His statement was based on an account provided by Dr. Norman Yoder, Commissioner of the Office of the Blind in the Pennsylvania State Welfare Department. Soon, however, the story was exposed as a hoax. On January 19, 1968, *The New York Times* reported that "the Governor, who yesterday told a news conference that he was convinced the report was true, said his investigators discovered this morning that the story was 'a fabrication' by Dr. Norman Yoder. . . . He said Dr. Yoder, who was unavailable for comment, had admitted the hoax. . . . Officials here were stunned by the Governor's announcement. They generally described Dr. Yoder as a selfless, well-liked, and reliable public servant."[17]

These disclosures had not the slightest effect either on the crusade against drug abuse or on Governor Shafer's standing as an expert on this subject. Dr. Yoder and his lies were disposed of by the method characteristic of our age. He was immediately categorized by Attorney General William C. Sennett as "distraught and sick," and his mendacity was attributed to "his concern over illegal LSD use by children."[18] These explanations hardly account for the enthusiastic acceptance of Dr. Yoder's story by the Pennsylvania state officials and the nation's press. The fact is that Dr. Yoder said what everyone wanted to hear and believe—namely, how terribly dangerous LSD really was.

Even after Dr. Yoder's story was branded a hoax by the Governor, a prominent Pennsylvania state senator insisted that it was true and that he had "evidence that the reported blinding of six college students during an LSD trance was not a hoax."[19] (Interestingly, Benjamin R. Donolow, the senator who made this claim, is a former narcotics agent.) Dr. Yoder remained unavailable to the press, having "entered the Philadelphia Psychiatric Center." To Senator Donolow, this meant that "Yoder was under intense pressure to identify the stricken students and may have decided to safeguard them and sacrifice his career by labeling his story a hoax. 'He's just the type of man to throw out a career to protect six kids,' Donolow said. 'He's a tremendous man of principle.' "[20]

None of this was mentioned, and I assume few people remembered it, when, in 1971, President Nixon appointed Raymond P. Shafer to the chairmanship of his newly organized Marijuana Commission. Perhaps even Governor Shafer himself forgot it all. In March 1972, when he held a news conference on the occasion of the issuing of the 1,184-page report of his Commission, he announced that "the time for politicizing the marijuana issue is at an end."[21] Did Governor Shafer believe this as sincerely as he did the fake story about the students blinded by staring at the sun?

Here, then, is the vexatious conclusion to which one is forced. If Governor Shafer believes that his report on marijuana is not political, then he is as sincerely deluded by his own ideology and mission as were the inquisitors who believed that their reports on the progress of the witch burnings were not religious but factual; and if he does not believe it, then he is asserting a deliberate falsehood.

I am making two simple points here. First, rabbis and priests, psychiatric and political drug experts, are not interested in, and do not tell us anything about, what *effects drugs* have; instead, they tell us how we should *conduct ourselves*. Second, whenever people tell us how to behave, we ought to evaluate the policy they recommend or prescribe by judging their grounds for it with the aid of observations and judgments other than those furnished by the policymakers themselves; if we do not, we have only ourselves to blame for the deception we thus invite.

Of course, I do not believe that there is such a thing as a "value-free" science, much less a value-free "social science." Hence, I do not urge anything so naïve as a value-free observer or observation; on the contrary, what I urge is that the observer's aims and values be as clear and explicit as possible. For example, it was clear to most Americans that Timothy Leary was not really interested in understanding how LSD works, but was interested rather in making people take it: he said so, and made money from saying so. It should be equally clear that persons who make a career out of prohibiting drugs are also not really interested in understanding how marijuana and heroin work, but are interested rather in preventing people from taking these drugs: some are honest enough to say so, and of course all of them make money from acting as if they said so. While there is no one who could be called neutral or disinterested in such a controversy, there are some—indeed, there are probably many—who refuse to proselytize for either the drug prohibitionists or the drug promoters.

It is sobering to note here that this very same phenomenon— that is, a party of prohibitionists opposed by a party of promoters,

neither of whose cause any self-respecting person could support—
had prevailed during Prohibition, and was duly remarked upon by
that great American observer of follies, public and private, Henry
Mencken. What Mencken had to say about this applies closely
to our present situation.

> Let us take a look, say, at the so-called drink problem, a small
> subdivision of the larger problem of saving men from their inherent
> and incurable hoggishness. What is the salient feature of the discus-
> sion of the drink problem, as one observes it going on eternally in
> These States? The salient feature of it is that very few honest and in-
> telligent men ever take a hand in the business—that the best men
> of the nation, distinguished for their sound sense in other fields, sel-
> dom show any interest in it. On the one hand it is labored by a horde
> of obvious jackasses, each confident that he can dispose of it over-
> night. And on the other hand it is sophisticated and obscured by a
> crowd of oblique fellows, hired by interested parties, whose secret
> desire is that it be kept unsolved. To one side, the professional gladi-
> ators of Prohibition; to the other side, the agents of the brewers
> and the distillers. But why do all neutral and clear-headed men
> avoid it? Why does one hear so little about it from those who have
> no personal stake in it, and can thus view it fairly and accurately?[22]

Mencken proposes several possible answers to this question,
only to dismiss them, and suggests that the reason why honest
and intelligent men stay clear of this "problem" is that "no genuinely intelligent man believes the thing is soluble at all."

I would add a further explanation of why intelligent people
avoid offering the sort of "analysis" of the alcohol—or drug—"problem" that Mencken was looking for, an explanation Mencken did
not mention because he did not view the problem as essentially
religious in character. If we so view it, the current drug controversy
comes to resemble the controversy between Catholics and Protestants during the heyday of the European religious wars. Two Christian sects were then pitted against each other. Some people
supported the Catholics, others the Protestants. Who could publicly undertake to scrutinize—and thus undermine—the beliefs and
mythologies of both? In such situations it is quite natural for some
persons to try to reinforce one set of ceremonial rules and mythological symbolizations, for others to try to reinforce the competing

set, and for those who are interested in demythologizing both sets to keep quiet.

The same considerations apply to our present situation. On the one hand, we have the Establishment, with its drug ceremonials and mythologies, and its powers to reward and punish; on the other side, we have the counter-culture, with its drug ceremonials and mythologies, and its powers to reward and punish. Thus, many politicians, physicians, and other "drug experts" now strive to reinforce the dominant drug mythologies and ceremonials; others —self-styled gurus and self-appointed scapegoats—strive to reinforce certain countervailing drug mythologies and ceremonials; still other persons—professionals and laymen alike—accept all drug mythologies and ceremonials for just what they are—and reject them all as scientific descriptions of chemical or pharmacological effects. And, as Mencken noted, those who support this third position—whatever their numbers—are conspicuous by their silence.

10. CURES AND CONTROLS: PANACEAS AND PANAPATHOGENS

Because one of the dominant passions of human beings is to control—themselves, other persons, and natural events—all cultures develop systems of explanations that function both as accounts of why good and bad things happen and as methods for causing them to happen. Magic and religion are, of course, the oldest and most familiar systems of such explanations and methods of control; or, more precisely, today, when we believe in science as an explanation and method of controlling persons and things, we *call* former beliefs and practices, in which we no longer believe, magical and religious.

In what follows, I shall not be concerned with the empirical validity of the claims attributed to the various "explanations" and "causes," as I shall consider only such extensions of them into explain-alls and cause-alls which are, at least to those who are not true believers in them, patently false. Indeed, the very concept of panacea implies such exaggerated powers—resembling powers that religions attribute to deities—as to engender doubt as well as faith. The *Oxford English Dictionary* defines a panacea as "a remedy, cure, or medicine, reputed to heal all diseases"; and it offers such examples of its use as the following: "Phlebotomie, which is their panacea for all diseases (1652)"; and "Coffee was his panacea (1867)."

The magical or religious character of panaceas—and of their opposites, which I shall call "panapathogens"—is also revealed by the role they have played and continue to play in the history of medicine. Simply put, these two categories of agents—formerly theological but now therapeutic in character—are the saviors and scapegoats of society; they constitute the ceremonial symbols for the collectivity's rituals of purification and pollution.[1] (For a list of the principal panaceas and panapathogens in the history of the Western world, see Table 2.)

Medicine has a dual social character and function: to cure disease and to control deviance. For far too long, however, the

TABLE 2
THE PRINCIPAL PANACEAS AND PANAPATHOGENS
IN THE HISTORY OF THE WESTERN WORLD

Period or World View	Panacea	Panapathogen
1. Christianity	God Baptism Jesus Imitation Faith Prayer Misery Benediction Resurrection Sacraments Holy water	Satan Original sin Jews Originality Skepticism Blasphemy Pleasure Malediction Insurrection Sacrilege Witch's brew
2. Enlightenment	Knowledge Science	Ignorance Superstition
3. 18th and 19th century medicine	Opium	Masturbation
4. Individualism	Freedom and responsibility	Determinism and planning
5. Collectivism	The state	The individual
6. Modern scientific-statist world view	Internationalism Science Research Innovation Physician	Nationalism Magic Religion Tradition Quack
7. Pharmacracy	Legitimate, "holy" drugs	Illegitimate, "unholy" drugs

doctor's role as priest or policeman has been subsumed under, and disguised as, his role as physician—with the unfortunate result that the relief of pain has become commingled and confused with the repression of protest, both being called simply "treatment."

I believe the time is ripe now for pinpointing the differences between these two radically disparate medical functions; that is, for identifying, accurately and honestly, the mechanisms—linguistic, legal, moral, and technical—by means of which the medical profession, at the behest of both the state and its own ambitions for power, exercises social control over personal conduct.

Inasmuch as we have words to describe medicine as a healing art, but have none to describe it as a method of social control or political rule, we must first give it a name. I propose that we call it *pharmacracy,* from the Greek roots *pharmakon,* for "medicine" or "drug," and *kratein,* for "to rule" or "to control." Pharmacology is the science of drugs, and especially of the therapeutic and toxic effects and uses of drugs. It is appropriate, then, that a system of political controls based on and exercised in the name of drugs should be called a "pharmacracy." As theocracy is rule by God or priests, and democracy is rule by the people or the majority, so pharmacracy is rule by medicine or physicians.

In the sense in which I propose to use this term, pharmacracy is the characteristic technical form of that particular modern socio-political organization which more than a decade ago I named the "Therapeutic State."[2] Contemporary pharmacracies rule mainly by means of drug controls—a rule aptly symbolized by the linguistic and legal powers of the physician's "prescription." Their rule is of relatively recent origin: it is sometime during the nineteenth century somewhere in western Europe—I have been unable to ascertain the exact time and place—that, for the first time in human history, the law distinguishes between ordinary citizen on the one hand and physician and pharmacist on the other, prohibiting the former from free access to certain "drugs," reserving such access, for the purpose of providing "treatment," to the latter.[3] We have since witnessed the steady growth of the powers of pharmacracy. Today especially in the United States, its rule is absolute and capricious—that is, tyrannical. Although pharmacracies now rule mainly by means of drug controls and psychiatric controls—that is, by using medical justifications and personnel for repressing "dangerous drugs" and "dangerous mental patients"—it is quite possible that as these methods are publicly exposed and thus rendered morally distasteful, the technology of pharmacratic repression may shift to behavior modification and psychosurgery.

In the modern Western therapeutic societies, the political and medical decision makers control the definition of drugs as therapeutic or toxic, and hence also their legitimacy and availability in the marketplace. The definitions of tobacco and alcohol as agricultural products and of marijuana and opium as dangerous drugs—definitions authenticated by both the United States government and the United Nations—at once illustrate that we live in a pharmacracy, and display its particular values.

The difference between pharmacology and pharmacracy—that is, between science as a body of facts and theories and scientism as a system of justifications for social policy and social control—is illustrated by the following typical account from the daily press. In an Associated Press report entitled "Saccharin Suspect in Study," the American people were informed—in the first sentence of the story—that "a new federal report shows 'presumptive evidence' that saccharin in high doses causes cancerous bladder tumors in rats."[4] What those who read the rest of the story discovered was that forty-eight rats were fed saccharin as 7.5 percent of their total diet and that three of these rats developed tumors that "may be" cancerous. Nowhere in the newspaper report, running to some three hundred words, was there even the merest hint that rats fed, for example, sodium chloride—that is, table salt—as 7.5 percent of their total diet might not remain very healthy either. Instead, the reader was told, in tones of high solemnity, that "the Food and Drug Administration said it will not move against saccharin, the only artificial sweetener remaining on the market since cyclamate was banned, until it received a recommendation from the National Academy of Sciences."[5]

When cigarettes were discovered to be toxic—something that had been known for decades before the "discovery" became officially recognized by the United States government—they were labeled as "dangerous to health." When cyclamate was discovered to be toxic—a claim whose validity, in cases where the substance is used in low doses, remains in serious doubt—it was banned entirely: pharmaceutical companies are enjoined from manufacturing it and people cannot buy it. Similarly, in the report cited above, the public is not told that, should saccharin prove to be potentially toxic, it would be so labeled; instead, it is told that, if the National Academy of Sciences "recommends" banning saccharin, then the government will ban it. That is pharmacracy in action.

Ostensibly, "therapeutic" panaceas are agents of medical cure; actually, they are—just as are those that are overtly religious—

agents of magical control. A brief review of some of the major "therapeutic" panaceas of the past two thousand years will support this interpretation, and show how remarkably similar the claims for these various agents actually are.

Galen (130–c. 200) was the founder of the most important school of medicine of his age, a school whose influence extended through the Middle Ages. In Galenic practice the most useful medicine was a *theriaca,* or antidote, named *Electuarium theriacale magnum,* a compound composed of several ingredients, among them opium and wine. Its powers, according to Galen, were as follows: "It resists poison and venomous bites, cures inveterate headache, vertigo, deafness, epilepsy, apoplexy, dimness of sight, loss of voice, asthma, coughs of all kinds, spitting of blood, tightness of breath, colic, the iliac poison, jaundice, hardness of the spleen, stone, urinary complaints, fevers, dropsies, leprosies, the troubles to which women are subject, melancholy, and all pestilences."[6]

Although opium remained a medical panacea until the end of the nineteenth century, from the Middle Ages on similar claims were made for other substances as well, especially for alcohol. Here is a thirteenth-century account of the beneficent powers of alcohol—which, of course, used to be called *aqua vitae,* the water of life:

> It sloweth age, it strengtheneth youth, it helpeth digestion, it abandoneth melancholie, it relisheth the heart, it lighteneth the mind, it quickeneth the spirit, it keepeth and preserveth the head from whirling, the eyes from dazzling, the tongue from lisping, the mouth from snaffling, the teeth from chattering, and the throat from rattling; it keepeth the stomach from wambling, the heart from swelling, the hands from shivering, the sinews from shrinking, the veins from crumbling, the bones from aching, and the marrow from soaking.[7]

In China, the medical panacea was tea. The following is a description of tea sold in Canton in the second half of the nineteenth century:

> The never-failing Midday Tea; its taste and odour are pure and fragrant, its qualities temperate and mild. . . . The stomach is

strengthened by its use; it creates appetite, dissolves secretions, assuages the most burning thirst, checks colds, dispels vapours; in a word, the inner distempers and outer complaints are all allayed by this tea. Is it not divine? . . . The medicinal herbs of which it is composed are culled with the nicest attention. . . . It is dared to be publicly asserted, that although it may not always be *positively* beneficial in illness, yet in respect to longevity it will be found wonderful.[8]

The language in which the claims for the evil effects of panapathogens are cast, and the imagery they conjure up, parallels the language and imagery of panaceas. Until the Renaissance the leading Western panapathogens were the devil, witches, and Jews. Since then, they have been madness, masturbation, and, most recently, dangerous drugs, addicts, and pushers.

The transformation of panaceas into panapathogens is both a cause and a consequence of the ideological transformation that it expresses. Although seemingly a radical change, such a transformation is often no more than a change in ceremonial symbols, leaving the basic fabric of social organization and control largely unaltered. For example, with the change in Russia from Czarism to Communism, the religious panaceas of Christianity become panapathogens; the oligarchic, tyrannical nature of Russian rule, however, remained the same. Similarly, with the change in medical sexology from Krafft-Ebing and Freud to Masters and Johnson, masturbation was transformed from panapathogen into panacea; the paternalistic rule of doctors over patients, however, remained the same.

This metamorphosis—for which the degradation of opium and cocaine are our best examples—progresses through a definite pattern of discrete phases. First, the substance—let us call it X—is freely available. As the rulers realize that, although X is not required for survival, people want it and will pay money for it, they seize upon it as a source of revenue: the government now imposes a tax on X, subjecting it to economic regulation. Next, X is defined as a drug, making its use legitimate only for the treatment of illness: the government, with the zealous support of the medical profession, now restricts its use to prescription by a physician, subjecting X to medical controls. This creates both a black market in X and "abuses" in its medical distribution through physicians' "overprescriptions," setting the stage for political and popular demand for more stringent controls over X. Finally, to justify and facilitate total prohibition, "medical research" reveals that there are no "legitimate therapeutic" indications or uses for X at all: since any and all use of X is now viewed as "abuse," politicians, physicians, and the people unite in banning X altogether.

We have actually lived through this pattern of escalating prohibition—transforming a freely available useful substance into the strictly prohibited scourge of mankind—with both opium and cocaine. We have lived through some of its phases, without carrying the process to completion, with alcohol, tobacco, amphetamines, vitamins A and D in large doses, and other substances. It seems safe to predict that in the near future we are likely to see other substances—perhaps aspirin, saccharin, and who knows what else—subjected to such pharmacratic controls. To help appreciate the influence of permissions, prescriptions, and prohibitions on our ideas about drugs and their uses, I have constructed, in Table 3, a classification of drugs—not, as is customary, in terms of their pharmacological actions, but in terms of their availability, distribution, and use.

Just as the human impulses to cure and to control are at once complementary and contradictory, so too are the principles of pharmacology and pharmacracy. I have indicated this relationship between them in Table 4. The idea of control is an all-inclusive concept, subsuming the notion of cure. Treatment, as we usually conceive of it, is a non-coercive type of social control, relying for its effect wholly on the initiative and cooperation of the sick person. Whereas contemporary drug laws (and mental hygiene and public health laws) are coercive types of social controls, relying for their effects on the police powers of the state. This interpretation is consistent with all our historical experience with medicine as a healing art.

Before the second half of the nineteenth century, when modern therapeutic medicine as we now know it took its first stumbling steps, there was virtually nothing that physicians could do to alleviate disease. And the less effective were their remedies, the

TABLE 3

A CLASSIFICATION OF DRUGS BY MODE OF AVAILABILITY, DISTRIBUTION, AND USE

Class of Drug	Exemplifying Members of the Class	Expected Use
I. Non-medical drugs ("Non-drugs")		
1. Foods	Sugar, carbohydrates, fats, and proteins	As part of "normal" diet
2. Substances added to foods	Salt, condiments and spices, food colorings, preservatives, other chemicals	As part of "normal" process of eating commercially merchandised foods
3. Beverages	Water, coffee, tea, cocoa, etc.	As part of "normal" diet
4. Substances added to water	Chlorine, fluorides, and other chemicals	As part of "normal" process of drinking "medically safe" water
5. Substances applied to the body	Cosmetics, perfumes, antiperspirants, etc.	As part of "normal" process of beautifying the body
6. Body cleansers	Soap, toothpaste, mouthwash, douches, etc.	As part of "normal" process of cleaning the body
7. Socially acceptable recreational substances	Alcohol, nicotine, caffeine	At all socially appropriate occasions and times
8. Substances used in the home, industry, transportation, etc.	Gasoline, detergents, lye, glue, paint, varnish, pesticides, furniture polish, etc.	As part of "normal" process of homemaking, farming, manufacturing, traveling, etc.
II. Medical drugs ("Therapeutic drugs")		
9. Over-the-counter drugs	Antacids Anti-cold medicines Aspirin Laxatives Vitamins	If slightly ill (diagnosed by self)
10. Prescription drugs	Insulin Morphine Penicillin	If seriously ill (diagnosed by physician)
11. Drugs restricted to special medical personnel and settings	Antabuse Methadone	If "specially" ill ("addict")
III. Illegal drugs		
12. Disapproved therapeutic drugs	Thalidomide	None
13. Disapproved food and beverage additives or substitutes	Cyclamates	None
14. Disapproved recreational drugs	Heroin Cocaine Marijuana	If member of counter-culture (if desires to defy the "establishment")

TABLE 4
CURE AND CONTROL

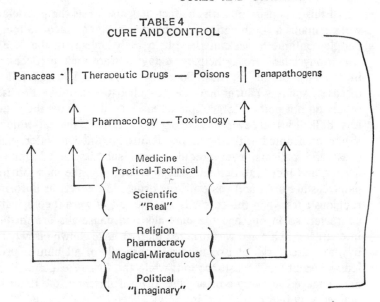

more plentiful were their panaceas: besides opium and alcohol, phlebotomy (bloodletting), purgation with calomel (mercurous chloride), blistering, and a host of other things that physicians gave to patients or did to them were all regarded, at one time or another, as cure-alls. Since the development of effective therapeutic agents and measures, especially during the past few decades, medical scientists and physicians have learned that every chemical and physical intervention in the human organism produces certain clear-cut consequences in it. Instead of panaceas or general remedies, physicians now speak of specific measures, useful for one or at most a few conditions, but useless or harmful for others. Penicillin is therapeutic for some infections, but not for others; an appendectomy is therapeutic only for an acutely inflamed appendix; and so forth. In contrast, such modern "medical treatments" as Christian Science, psychoanalysis, the mud and waters of spas, vegetarianism, and vitamin C reveal their characters as panaceas through their alleged powers to prevent and cure an almost endless variety of ailments.

All this is consistent with the fact that insofar as the physician's work remains a combination of applied science and medical magic, people continue to seek medical help for problems in the face of which physicians are as helpless today as were their predecessors in the face of the plagues. Some of these problems pertain to diseases, such as cancer and the so-called degenerative diseases; others do not pertain to genuine diseases at all, such as the countless difficulties of everyday living now called "mental illness." When confronted with these, physicians continue to offer panaceas; and patients, ever credulous and submissive, continue to accept, and indeed to demand, them. In our day, the most obvious panaceas are diets and tranquilizing drugs. Moreover, as in former religious ages when the cure-alls and cause-alls were theological in character, so in our age the cure-alls and cause-alls are medical in character. This age was ushered in, as I have shown elsewhere,[9] by the "discovery" of two medical cause-alls of all human problems: insanity and masturbation; while the former explained why men engaged in every conceivable form of mischief, the latter explained why they contracted insanity!

Although it is now nearly three hundred years old, the concept of mental illness—as a panchreston (explain-all) and panapathogen—has reached its full flowering only in our day; with its efflorescence, there have emerged special instances or members of it, such as drug abuse and drug addiction—the causes and symptoms of mental illness in the Free Societies; and religious observances—the causes and symptoms of mental illness in the Communist Societies.

To be sure, the Communists don't like narcotics either. They are against all sorts of things which express or symbolize the autonomy of the individual. My point, however, is that just as our principal panapathogen now is the Dangerous Drug, the Communists' is the Dangerous Religion. If this parallel—and more specifically, the parallel between heroin and holy water—seems exaggerated, perhaps the following report, distributed by the Associated Press, will make it seem less so.

On March 27, 1973, "an Austrian Catholic news service reported that a priest, identified as Stephan Kurti, had been executed in Albania, condemned to death for secretly baptizing a child."[10]

Evidently, to the Albanians, Kurti is a "pusher" of holy water who deserves to die, just as to many Americans, importers of heroin are "pushers" who also deserve to die.

Moreover, just as the Capitalist Crusade is aimed not only against heroin but against all "dangerous drugs," so the Communist Crusade is aimed not only against holy water but against all religions.

From the same Associated Press report we learn that, on March 31, 1973, the Vatican radio announced that Communist Albania " 'has suffocated all forms of Christian life in its plan aimed at the total destruction of the Roman Catholic Church. . . . There are no religious buildings. . . . They have all been transformed into dance halls, gymnasiums, or government offices. . . . The Orthodox churches and the Moslem mosques had the same fate.' "[11]

This is not an isolated report. Other Communist authorities on mental health have long claimed that religion causes countless mental diseases and social disorders, a claim identical to that which American mental health experts make about "dangerous drugs." For example, according to a 1972 Associated Press news report from Prague, the Slovak Communist party organ *Pravda* has warned "Czechoslovak parents . . . that religion constitutes a grave hazard for the mental health of children. Religion interferes with sound and harmonious emotional development . . . it impedes social adaptability, creating the conditions for the emergence of delinquency. By burdening the nervous system, it leads to psychical disorders. It brings up individuals with an undermined will and stands in the way of the development of firm moral sentiments. . . . It weakens the will to learn, leading to lower grades."[12]

This Communist image of religion as panapathogen is just as much a part of their customs and laws as our image is concerning drugs: we warn travelers not to bring narcotics into the United States; the Russians warn travelers not to bring Bibles into the U.S.S.R.[13]

These examples amply demonstrate that the differences between pharmacology and pharmacracy are, in the last analysis, the same as the differences between description and prescription, fact and value, medicine and morals. In short, panaceas and panapathogens are counters in a calculus of justificatory rhetoric: they do not assert facts, but justify—nay, incite to—actions.

Although ostensibly aimed at protecting the layman, pharmacratic controls ultimately injure both patient and physician. The citizen as potential sick person is injured because he is deprived of the right to self-medication; of the opportunity and right to select the expert of his choice—some experts being declared unlicensed and thus prevented by law from offering their services; and of the right to treatment with certain drugs which, although available in other countries, may be forbidden in the United States, even through prescription by accredited physicians.[14]

The physician, favored in the short run by such controls as the beneficiary of a government-protected monopoly, is ultimately also victimized, mainly as a result of the enforcement of precisely those drug controls whose ostensible aim was only the protection of uninformed laymen from "using the wrong medicine." This seemingly altruistic motive and practical goal conceals the drive for domination—of patient by physician, of some physicians by others, of physician by politician, in an unending spiral of regulations and tyrannizations.

The upshot is that the physician is no longer free to prescribe the drug he believes would most benefit his patient, as he was twenty or fifty years ago. First, because he fears that if he prescribes certain drugs, especially psychoactive drugs, "too often" or in quantities considered to be "excessive"—so judged by committees of his peers—he may be punished by sanctions ranging from reprimands to loss of his license to practice medicine.[15] Further, because he fears that since copies of his prescription of "controlled substances" go on file in centralized, politicized registries, these records might later be used to injure his patient —legally, economically, occupationally, or in ways now impossible to anticipate.[16] Lastly, because he fears—or ought to fear—that the person seeking his help is not a patient at all, but an *agent provocateur*. I refer here to an aspect of the war on drugs that has been completely concealed from the public and hence deserves more detailed comment.

Judging by the citation of legal decisions, it has evidently been common law enforcement practice in recent years to deploy undercover narcotics agents posing as patients to doctors' offices, to entrap physicians into prescribing "controlled substances" illegally. Here are the summaries of two such cases, culled from the American Medical Association's periodical abstract of judicial decisions.

In the first case, "an undercover agent assigned to conduct an investigation of illegal narcotic traffic went to the physician's office posing as a patient. He told the physician he was suffering from the aftereffects of taking mescaline and that he was nervous and having trouble sleeping."[17] Perhaps medical schools and textbooks should expand the scope of their instruction: they teach the student about "addicts" and "malingerers," but do not teach him about *agents provocateurs*—now called "narcotics agents"—who "pose as patients," fake symptoms and diseases, and seek to entrap the physician into prescribing or dispensing drugs illegally.

The physician in the above case gave the "patient" some barbiturate pills. "The agent returned to the physician's office five more times, requesting prescriptions. . . ." Each time, the physician, a woman, complied—with the result that she "was found guilty of 13 indictments charging violations of various narcotic drug statutes and regulations." In court, the physician argued the defense of entrapment, but the jury ruled against her. She appealed, contending that "it had not been proved beyond a reasonable doubt that she did not act in good faith and that the amount of drugs dispensed was excessive. . . . The court said the evidence was sufficient to warrant the jury's conclusion that the physician did not act in good faith and that dispensing to the agent of any quantity of drugs or narcotics was excessive and impelled by no legitimate medical purpose. The court said the jury could reach its conclusions from the physician's conduct and testimony, unassisted by expert testimony."[18]

The story speaks for itself. I want to note only that what is a "legitimate medical purpose" for prescribing narcotics was here determined by a jury of non-physicians. The physicians who have so zealously supported the war on "dangerous drugs" no doubt never anticipated that this would be one of its consequences.

In another case, a special agent of the Bureau of Narcotics and Dangerous Drugs "visited a physician in his office and complained of a persistent backache. Without conducting a physical examination, the physician prescribed Parafon Forte."[19] After more compromising behavior with this agent, a second agent was deployed to entrap the doctor. This pseudo-patient "complained of nervousness and inability to sleep." The physician "prescribed Librium, again without conducting a physical examination." This agent also returned for subsequent visits, and obtained more drugs. The physician was convicted "on two counts of improperly prescribing controlled drugs to agents of the Federal Bureau of Narcotics and Dangerous Drugs." His conviction was affirmed by a federal appellate court.[20]

This account also speaks for itself. Here I would like to add, however, that psychiatrists regularly prescribe "controlled substances" to patients they do not physically examine. In fact, many psychiatrists believe that it is improper for a physician to examine physically a patient whom he is "treating" by psychotherapy; yet many of these psychiatrists prescribe drugs for their patients. Is the conduct of all of these physicians in violation of the rules and regulations of the Federal Bureau of Narcotics and Dangerous Drugs?

The Harrison Act, passed in 1914, aimed ostensibly at controlling addicts, was actually used to control physicians. That act, it should be recalled, criminalized the free, over-the-counter sale of opium and its derivatives, and made these drugs legally available only through a physician's prescription for the treatment of disease. In a series of Supreme Court decisions following the passage of the act, the Court declared that dispensing or prescribing opiates to addicts is outside the scope of legitimate medical practice and therefore also illegal. According to a study sponsored by the New York Academy of Medicine, in the years following the passage of the Harrison Act, and especially after 1919, 25,000 physicians were arraigned on charges of selling narcotics, and 3,000 actually served prison sentences. Thousands more had their licenses revoked.[21] The handwriting was on the wall, but the American medical profession stubbornly refused to read it.

I have discussed elsewhere the grievous violations committed by physicians against the freedom and dignity of so-called mental patients; in those cases, the protections of the rule of law of a free society are abandoned in favor of the madness controls promised by a tyrannous pharmacracy. Here I want to expose and denounce the grievous violations committed by politicians, legislators, and jurists against the freedom and dignity of physicians; in these cases, the protections of the rule of law of a free society are abandoned in favor of the drug controls promised by a tyrannous pharmacracy.

Threatened with plagues and famines, the medieval European set out to solve his problems by persecuting witches and Jews. Threatened with imperialistic Communism, a shortage of energy, and environmental pollution, the modern American sets out to solve his problems by persecuting marijuana smokers and heroin sellers.

In the American temper, moreover, the panapathogen must not only be combated in action but, perhaps more importantly, must also be legislated out of existence. In 1971, in the Commonwealth of Massachusetts alone, some 143 bills relating to drugs have been introduced. One of these provides for the death penalty "for the possession of with intent to sell narcotic drugs." If all these bills were passed, notes the *Massachusetts Physician,* "a person carrying aspirin tablets might be in jeopardy."[22]

It is indeed tragic that physicians, and people generally, should remain so blind to the wisdom of the Gospels and delude themselves that they can ignore with impunity Jesus' warning that ". . . all who take the sword shall perish by the sword";[23] that, in other words, all who plan, promote, and profit from drug controls shall perish from drug controls.

Such a warning as this comes, of course, too late to save "free" American medicine from the government controls that threaten it, as American medicine has for too long been a government monopoly rather than a free profession. However, my adaptation, to the requirements of the contemporary drug scene, of a time-honored wisdom from the Gospels makes a fitting epitaph for the headstone of a Medicine devoted to curing the sick but murdered by a brother devoted to controlling the sinful.

11. TEMPTATION AND TEMPERANCE: THE MORAL PERSPECTIVE RECONSIDERED

While the impact of the change from a religious to a scientific world-view on people's relations to their non-human environment is well appreciated, its impact on their relations to themselves and to their fellow human beings remains poorly, and even incorrectly, understood. The reason for this lies, in my opinion, in the very nature of science.

The essence of the scientific enterprise is the effort to understand something the better to control it. In natural science, this means that the scientist, a person, studies and controls the object of his interest, a thing. The thing studied has no say in this matter. Hence the moral dimensions and dilemmas of natural science derive not from a conflict between the scientist and the object he studies, but from a conflict between the scientist and other persons or groups who may disapprove of the personal and social consequences of his work.

In human or moral "science" the situation is radically different. Here, the scientist, a person, studies and controls the object of his interest, another person. The subject studied is very much concerned with this process. Hence, the moral dimensions and dilemmas of human science derive from two distinct sources: first, from a conflict between the scientist and the subject, and second, from a conflict between the scientist and other persons or groups who may disapprove of the personal and social consequences of his work.

Thus, although both the natural and moral sciences seek to understand the objects of their observation, in natural science the purpose of this is to be able to control them better, whereas in moral science it is, or ought to be, to be better able to leave them alone. In my opinion, the only morally proper aim of psychology can be to maximize personal self-control.

This, of course, is not the way the task of psychology, psychiatry, or the other social "sciences" is usually interpreted. On the contrary, their nature and task are seen as analogous to those of the natural sciences—that is, as the study, prediction, and control of human behavior.

The reason for this link between science and social control, between technology and totalitarianism, lies simply in the fact that human behavior can be controlled in two ways, and two ways only: by the person himself, through self-control; or by another person (or group), through coercion. *Tertium non datur;* there is no third way.

It follows that the more man's view of human nature emphasizes spiritual values, free will, and human differentiation and self-determination, the greater will be the scope of controlling conduct through self-control. And the more man's view of human nature emphasizes material values, scientific determinism, and human equality and perfectibility, the greater will be the scope of controlling conduct through external coercion. Science is thus as well-suited to perfecting interpersonal coercion as religion had been to perfecting personal asceticism.

If left unchecked by countervailing considerations, each of these ideologies leads to death and destruction in the name of "liberation." In his unrestrained pursuit of self-control, the ascetic abstains from food and water, sex and speech, clothing and comfort, to find "freedom" in personal dissolution. While in his unrestrained pursuit of control over others, the true believer in "scientific humanism" (or by whatever name he chooses to call his creed) overshoots his mark in the opposite direction. Since his self-appointed task is to make the other "healthy" and "happy," and since, as he is bound to discover, he is frustrated in achieving this task by what he regards as his "patient's" inadequate or improper self-control, he sets himself to reducing, and ultimately eliminating, his self-control. The result is, again, death: physical death, through the liquidation of those who resist the interventions of the authorities whose credo is: "Be happy, or die!"; and spiritual death—in the ways forecast and described by Zamiatin, Huxley, and Orwell—through the robotization of those who comply with the authorities.

Actually, man had, in the past, placed various, and generally satisfactory, restraints on his overzealousness toward controlling himself—restraints which need not concern us here. He now places various restraints on his overzealousness toward controlling others—restraints which are, and should be, of serious concern to everyone who values freedom and dignity today. Among these restraints, the following seem to me the most significant.

The more insistently the "scientists" assert that "people"—that is, their subjects—have no free will, the more tightly they back them into a corner where the people must ask whether the "scientists"—that is, their actual or would-be rulers—have or do not have free will. And if they do not, who determines or controls their choices? We recognize in this dilemma a secular re-enactment of the religious dilemma posed by the divine rights of rulers: either they had to accept their rulers as literal divinities; or they had to confront the possibility that their rulers were only metaphorically divine, while actually they were human. The mythology of scientific determinism in human affairs suffers from exactly the same logical weakness; it is a quite satisfactory justification of authority for people who are true believers in the *religion of science*—but *only* for them.

Another restraint on man's passion to control his fellow man derives from what seems to be a characteristic of "human nature," perhaps its most "divine" characteristic—namely, the tendency for efforts to control people to generate an equally strong resistance in the subjects to reject the control, often by acting in a direction counter to that in which they are coerced. Innumerable relationships between people, and even between people and things, illustrate this principle. Among the latter, I am especially fond of this one, which seems to me a veritable scientific parable: To hold a wet bar of soap securely, one must grasp it lightly; the harder one squeezes it, the more likely it is to slip out of one's grasp.

In human relations one need hardly cite examples to illustrate the principle that coercion stimulates resistance, prohibition engenders desire. It is not merely that forbidden fruit tastes sweeter, but rather that the very act of forbidding makes a previously neutral act "sweet." The reason for this is not hard to discern. It is mainly by resisting authority that the individual defines himself. This is why authorities—whether parental, priestly, political, or psychiatric—must be careful how and where they assert themselves; for while it is true that the more they assert themselves the more they govern, it is also true that the more they assert themselves the more opportunities they offer for being successfully defied. The maxim "He who governs least, governs best" not only expresses the basic principle of decency and dignity in statecraft; it also furnishes the only preventive known to mankind against the characteristic crowd madnesses of overcontrol, manifested by the war on witchcraft formerly and by the war on drugcraft today.

One of the most serious and most tragic consequences of the contemporary secularized-technical view on drug taking, drug giving, and drug avoiding is the blindness it engenders toward what is, in my opinion, the single most important theme in this drama—namely, the struggle against temptation and the surrender to it.

The theme of temptation is as ancient as recorded civilization. It is present in all religions, even the most primitive, and in all systems of ethics. And it plays a central, though today largely unacknowledged, role in all systems of healing, especially in those of contemporary psychiatry.

Furthermore, we cannot understand temptation unless we understand sacrifice: each is the reciprocal of the other. Sacrifice is the deliberate, voluntary renunciation of a possession, a pleasure, or a power. Originally, man engages in the sacrificial act vis-à-vis a supernatural power or deity and, through the sacrifice, transforms something ordinary or profane into something holy or sacred.[1] Primitive man thus sacrifices his most valued possessions —domestic animals and other foodstuffs—to the gods.

To understand the significance of sacrifice, we must recognize its several meanings: it is a ceremonial acknowledgment of the authority of God and man's willing subjection to Him; it is an act of atonement for sins and a symbolic restitution for misdeeds; and —most importantly from the point of view of our present interests —it is an affirmation of man's powers of self-control. By a deliberate and voluntary act of sacrifice—through one of those seeming paradoxes that characterize human nature and existence— the individual increases his control over himself. Emerson has put it perfectly: "We gain the strength of the temptation we resist."[2]

By acquiring self-control, man frees himself from the laws of reflexive subjection to needs, pleasures, and temptations. The farther a person carries this process of self-abnegation, the more successfully he overcomes or "denies" his "animal nature"—the more unlike an animal and the more like a "god" he becomes. Here lies the simple but inescapable connection between sacrifice, asceticism, "saintliness," self-control, and a sense of power over oneself—and sometimes an accompanying actuality of acquisition of power over others. And here lies the reciprocal connection between temptation, yielding to temptation, self-indulgence, weakness, and a sense of loss of control over oneself—and often an accompanying actuality of loss of power over others.

To offer a sacrifice, man must possess something whose loss would give him pain and whose voluntary renunciation therefore constitutes a sacrifice. Whereas to be tempted, he must lack something whose acquisition would give him pleasure and whose voluntary acceptance therefore constitutes yielding to temptation. Hence it is that the possibilities for sacrifice and pain are so much richer than those for temptation and pleasure. For the possibilities for temptation actually come down to a few types, which are only all too familiar from biblical and other mythological sources.

First, there is the temptation represented by the Serpent and by Eve—that is, the temptation to "know" either the spirit or the flesh, to satisfy curiosity or lust. There are hints here to the relations, in the human being, between cognition and carnal "knowledge" that I will not consider. Second, there is the temptation, represented in the symbol of the Tower of Babel, of cooperation among persons and of the power they can so gain. The lure of power, however, is expressed more directly and clearly in the devil's tempting of Jesus in the desert by offering Him the kingdom of earth. Finally, there is the temptation of the flesh, of erotic voluptuousness, familiar to us through the countless temptresses from Delilah and Salome to Lorelei and the modern "sex goddesses."

In short, most temptations fall into one of the following classes: knowledge, power, and sex. It is significant that the lure of drugs is not among the temptations dramatized in either pagan or Christian mythology, an omission that cannot be attributed to the absence of what we now consider addictive drugs: people have been familiar with alcohol, marijuana, and opiates during the very epochs when the mythologies of temptation I have just reviewed originated and dominated the minds of men. The "pleasures" that drugs offer are thus of a different kind than are the satisfactions of those human drives that form the themes of classic accounts of temptation.

To understand our present attitude toward drugs, it is necessary to understand the traditional (religious) position on temptation and to appreciate its similarities with, and differences from, the modern (secular) position on it.

In the Christian ethic, man's ability to resist temptation is roughly the measure of his virtuousness in the eye of God. This is why the temperate person is its ideal, and the ascetic—the champion at resisting temptation—is its hero. Of course, this principle can be "abused" too: resistance to temptation, which is a means to an end, namely salvation, can become an end in itself. In making renunciation the goal of life, man succumbs to the temptation to reject all temptation, once and for all time.

With the dissolution of the religious world-view which began during the Renaissance and Enlightenment, this whole perspective on seduction, sacrifice, and self-control underwent a profound change. As often happens when a moral value is rejected, the path of least resistance lies in embracing its opposite: If sacrifice is rejected, the hoarding of goods becomes exalted. Thus the vice of temptation becomes the virtue of advertising; the strength of self-control becomes the sickness of self-inhibition; and the weakness of surrender becomes the reasonableness of rational man capable of compromise and of the responsiveness of a "virile" man capable of "loving" a "feminine" woman.

A few aphorisms and proverbs will illustrate this transformation—from a religious to a secular, from a spiritual to a scientific perspective. "Temperance," Cicero observes, "consists in forgoing bodily pleasures."[3] A Latin proverb admonishes that "temperance is the best medicine."[4] The Bible teaches a similar lesson: "Blessed is the man that endureth temptation."[5] The perfect aphorism on the modern, "scientific" view of temptation is Oscar Wilde's recommendation: "The only way to get rid of a temptation is to yield to it."[6] Wilde here captures an all-important "truth"—provided that "free will" does not exist, and that self-control is at best a necessary illusion.

The subject of temptation and sacrifice appears, of course, in quite different guises today than it did in former, especially ancient, times. Indeed, as I shall presently show, we now lack a proper vocabulary for this subject. Before we can talk about it again, we shall first have to translate our current technical terms into their traditional moral equivalents. In short, we do not recognize temptations today because we have no words for them; and we have no words for them because we do not want to deal with them *as* temptations. For example, when people lure us to buy countless things that may or may not make our lives "better," we do not speak of "temptations"; and we call those who tempt us "advertisers." When we are offered drugs that our "betters" think are bad for us, we again do not speak of temptations; and we call those who tempt us "pushers." Our vocabulary thus precludes our seeing, much less confronting, the so-called drug problem as a problem of temptation and self-control.[7]

With this "scientific" degrading and devaluing of personal renunciation, sacrifice, and self-control, there develops a corresponding exaltation of the rights, and indeed the duties, of the community, or the state, to control not only the individual's conduct (which it always did) but also his passions (which it never did so long as religions were meaningful; the very attempt would have been senseless!).

The result, as René Gillouin has so well put it, is that "humanity no longer knows what temptation is. . . ."[8] Nowhere, I think, is this startling truth more powerfully evident than in the contemporary attitude toward the so-called problem of drug abuse and drug addiction. And nowhere is this truth more completely ignored. For although it is evident that drug abuse and drug addiction involve us in human situations in which no one is compelled, by external force, to take a drug—which makes the taking of illicit drugs, in part at least, clearly a matter of temptation and surrender to temptation—no modern "scientific" approach to this problem takes any account whatever of these concepts. Nor can it. Having reduced man to a biological organism, science—"behavioral science"--stands impotent before man the spiritual being.

With the transformation of the religious perspective on man into the scientific, and in particular into the psychiatric, which became fully articulated during the nineteenth century, there occurred a radical shift in emphasis away from viewing man as a *responsible agent acting in and on the world* and toward viewing him as a *responsive organism being acted upon by biological and social "forces."* In this process, the imagery and vocabulary of morality were replaced by biological fantasy and psychiatric metaphor. Temptation—resisted or indulged—has been supplanted by drives, instincts, and impulses—satisfied or frustrated. Virtue and vice have been transformed into health and illness. Thus, most so-called mental or psychiatric diagnoses actually refer to a person's conduct which is unconventional and unacceptable either because of what he is or is not tempted by, or because of the way he resists or yields to temptation.

One of the gravest psychiatric concerns in the nineteenth century was masturbation; and one of the most serious mental diseases was the madness it caused, namely "masturbatory insanity."[9] We saw how, in the psychiatric conceptualization of this behavior and the "illness" it "caused," what had formerly been the "temptation to masturbate" became the "impulse" to do so; and how the themes of resisting or yielding to temptation accordingly became the themes of possessing or lacking the strength to control the impulse. Yielding to temptation thus became the "symptom" of a lack in the personality or self (later in the ego!), this lack being interpreted as constituting a "mental disease." The result was the "manufacture" not only of masturbatory insanity but of all the so-called mental diseases characterized by what psychiatrists regarded as "impulsive behavior," such as "psychopathy." Nor did the psychiatric conquest of conduct stop here.

Although in some cases the new psychiatric standards of proper behavior were much the same as the previous religious standards had been, this was not always the case. For example, the temptation to engage in homosexual (or other prohibited sexual) acts was recognized in the Judeo-Christian ethic as a temptation—indeed, as a sexual temptation *more evil* than others and hence all the more strongly to be resisted. When biological, medical, and psychiatric codes replaced the religious ones, sexual deviations became much more intensely repudiated than they had ever been. This was an inevitable consequence of the medical perspective from which homosexuality came to be viewed: it could now no longer be regarded as a temptation—to be resisted like any other; instead, it had to be regarded as a temptation which a "normal" person simply would not have at all! Thus, those who engaged in homosexual conduct were "mentally sick" because they were overt homosexuals; and those who entertained such thoughts, or who were thought to entertain such thoughts by their psychoanalysts, were mentally sick because they were "latent homosexuals." In short, what had been "unnatural acts" or "acts against nature" in the religious perspective, became, in psychiatric terminology, "perverted" acts or "perverse" inclinations.

The medical and psychiatric standards of behavior that replaced the Judeo-Christian ones did not, however, simply relabel all of the old religious rules with new medical names. To be sure, some of the old rules were continued under new rubrics, at least for a while—for example, the prohibitions against homosexuality, adultery, theft, and murder. Others, however, were rejected, and were replaced by their very opposites. This was the case generally with respect to heterosexual genital activity. Whereas in the Christian ethic, sexual abstinence was the highest ideal, marital sexuality being allowed only as a concession to the needs of procreation, in the modern psychiatric ethic, sexual activity (of some types, between some partners) became a virtue (health) and sexual abstinence a vice (illness). This was particularly true for heterosexual genital activity, and especially in marriage. Thus, a man not tempted by a woman, especially his wife, or who resisted her sexual charms, was now said to be "impotent," and this condition was considered to be a form of mental disease. Similarly, the woman who was not tempted by the man or who resisted his charms, especially if he was her husband, was now said to be "frigid"; and this condition too was considered to be a form of mental disease. In this way a whole host of new "diseases" came into being, all of which had in common the fact that the person said to have been sick was not tempted, when, according to psychiatric standards, he should have been tempted; or if he was tempted, he refused to yield to it, when, according to psychiatric standards, he should have yielded.

Similarly, psychiatrists consider the male homosexual sick because he is not aroused by women, but is by men; consider the male heterosexual sick if he abstains from sexual activity, because he does not yield to a temptation to which he should; and consider men and women who gamble and lose their money sick, because they do not resist a temptation which they should. This list could easily be expanded, of course, as it includes all those "diseases" about which psychiatrists now speak or theorize in terms of "impulse disorders," "sexual disorders," "psychopathy," "delinquency," "acting out," "inhibitions," and "repressions."

This conceptual, moral, and semantic transformation from a religious to a medical world-view had to become reasonably well advanced before the "diseases" of drug abuse and drug addiction could be "discovered." For people have used and avoided drugs—and especially drugs that affect behavior—during all of recorded history. All this time it never occurred to anyone to regard another person who uses drugs differently than he does as "sick" —any more than it would have occurred to anyone to regard someone who worshipped differently as "sick." Of course, in former times no less than today, people possessed adequate means for demeaning or destroying those who disagreed with them or who defied their customs or laws. My point here is that these means were not medical or scientific, but religious and legal.

The cleric's traditional solution for all human problems (and even for many natural catastrophes) was to urge his parishioner to make ever-greater efforts at self-control. Sexual temptation, political oppression, economic privation, interpersonal conflict, disease—the "answer" to each was telling the sufferer to "turn the other cheek," "buck up," "snap out of it," or "take it like a man."

Where the clinician has not simply appropriated and renamed the cleric's ideas and interventions, he has inverted them—which is what he has done with respect to drug abuse and obesity: the "moralistic" message was to exaggerate the worth of self-control; the "medicalistic" message is to emphasize its utter worthlessness. The wonder cures for all the countless human problems are thus not moral but technical and, especially, medical. To be relieved of his suffering, the patient need not exert himself in any way; indeed, he need not do *anything,* except deliver himself, preferably without reservations, into the hands of the expert. This is why modern medical solutions for human problems resemble so closely the solutions of totalitarian politics, and why each comes to the same thing in the end: namely, to the exaltation of the state and its secular-religious agencies of social control—science, medicine, and especially psychiatry; and to the degradation of the individual to the status of a fibroblast in the metaphorical body politic of society. One could cite many examples to illustrate this downplaying by all contemporary "scientific" authorities of self-control as an appropriate means of regulating temptation. I shall cite three, each from a quite different authority and source.

One of the books that never lost its place on the best-seller list during the 1972–73 season was *Dr. Atkins' Diet Revolution.* Its author, Dr. Robert C. Atkins, a graduate of Cornell Medical School and a practicing internist, has, it seems, an exceptionally fine understanding of the real implications of medicine as a form of religion—and, in particular, of the idea that just as, in the Judeo-Christian ethic, self-control is a great virtue, so, in the medical ethic, it is a great vice. Accordingly, Atkins does not merely assert that "calories don't count": that, after all, has not only been said before, and with huge success, but also suffers from dignifying calories as still "relevant." Atkins is "not interested" in calories. The crux of his "revolution" is his unqualified hostility to "willpower"! Since the so-called obese person—who in actuality is often "addicted" not to food, but to dieting as a symbolic ritualization of inadequate willpower—feels that he lacks control over his weight and hence over himself, Atkins promises to give him complete control if he would only decide to reject self-control altogether. In effect, Atkins peddles the classic Grand Inquisitorial promise of offering people complete freedom if they would only first become complete slaves. The wording of a full-page advertisement for Dr. Atkins' book displays this message in its unconcealed splendor: "You can now command [*sic*] your body to Melt Away Fat" reads the top line in large print. The person who can't even command himself to eat less is assured that he can "command" his "body" to "melt away fat." Three lines down we come to the most revealing part of the message: "You don't need pills—you don't count calories—you don't even need willpower (because you're never hungry)!" The absence of hunger and hence—for those who follow Dr. Atkins' diet—the superfluity of willpower are then repeated on and off through the rest of the page.[10]

In short, Atkins promises complete relief from temptation, and complete conquest over it—for those who submit completely to him (or at least who buy his book). There are, of course, only three ways in which temptation may be controlled: by resisting it; by yielding to it; and by submission to external authority who will "regulate" its intensity and will otherwise "protect" one from it. Politicians and physicians are now united in urging the third option on mankind.

The source of my second example is the *American Medical News,* the weekly newspaper of the American Medical Association. In its November 27, 1972, issue, this publication reviewed a book on its first page, space not usually devoted to book reviews. The work so honored was edited by two physicians, David E. Smith, M.D., and George R. Gray, M.D. Its message—a message the American Medical Association now so enthusiastically endorses—is well expressed by its title, *It's So Good, Don't Even Try It Once.* The subtitle is more humorous because it is more mendacious: *Heroin in Perspective.* I shall not belabor this image of an irresistible temptation creating an irresistible impulse in an irresistibly stupid worshipper at the altar of the Church of American (or, for that matter, World) Medicine.

My final illustration will show that membership in this Church extends to all classes and races, all occupations and professions. Among its most blindly faithful adherents is William O. Douglas, widely considered to be one of the most "liberal" of our Supreme

Court Justices. In a landmark decision of the Court holding that "addiction" is a disease rather than a crime, Justice Douglas proclaimed the following "facts" about "addiction": "The addict is under compulsion not capable of managing without outside help. . . . We do know that there is a 'hard core' of chronic and incurable drug addicts who, in reality, have lost their power of self-control."[11] Nor is Douglas' "knowledge" limited to the nature of addiction; he also knows its cause, or possible origin: "The first step toward addiction may be as innocent as a boy's puff on a cigarette in an alleyway."[12]

I contend that Douglas says this, not because it is true, but because he wants to believe that it is. Anyone who smokes or drinks, or knows anyone who does, knows how much effort and practice it takes to learn to enjoy smoking cigarettes or drinking .martinis. Even Peter Laurie, a British journalist and author of one of the many typically contemporary and quite ordinary books on drugs, knows better and has the courage to say so. In a section appropriately titled "The Myths of Inevitable Addiction and the Pusher," he writes: "Addiction must, in fact, be the result of continued, conscious action, with some deterrents to be overcome like vomiting, the unpleasantness of sticking needles into veins, the expense and trouble of buying the drug on the black market. . . . 'It all became a bore. You have to work at being an addict,' says one who gave it up."[13]

Nevertheless, here is Douglas, who contemptuously rejects the "domino theory" of the Communist threat, but who wholeheartedly embraces the same "domino theory" when it is advanced by the World Church of Medicine to explain "addiction" and to justify controlling "addicts."

Actually, in his credulous belief in drugcraft, Douglas is resurrecting—whether he knows it or not—the mythology of masturbatory insanity: as a single act of masturbation was believed to lead, through an irresistible temptation to repeat it, to uncontrolled and uncontrollable masturbation and thence to insanity—so a single puff on a marijuana cigarette is now believed to lead, through an irresistible temptation to repeat it, to uncontrollable and uncontrolled craving for every "dangerous drug" in the pharmacopoeia, and thence to "incurable addiction." Such is the path of progress in epithetic psychiatry and in the "progressive" jurisprudence whose "liberal" decisions it informs.

These examples could, of course, be multiplied *ad infinitum*. Every newspaper and magazine, every radio and television program—not to mention the many "scientific" books on psychology and psychiatry, drugs and obesity, and so forth—work and rework this anti-self-control message. The gist of this message can be easily summarized: all mention or reference to self-discipline must be degraded and dismissed as "moralistic" and "unscientific"; and the most absurd ideas concerning man's complete helplessness to control himself and the most abhorrent methods to control him by external force must be extolled as "scientific" and "therapeutic."

In the modern "scientific" view of man, the notion of temptation thus occupies a curious place. Insofar as temptation relates to the person who is tempted, it is ignored, eliminated, or transformed into something objective, "scientific"—almost tangible and quantifiable: temptation becomes a "force" to which a person "gives in" or under which he "breaks." The mechanical metaphor of a plank or bridge giving way under a heavy load replaces the moral metaphor of man resisting or yielding to evil. This is consistent with the deterministic, "scientific" view of man, according to which there is no soul, no free will, and of course no good and evil.

We do not—and cannot—expect a bridge built to sustain a five-ton load to "buck up" and carry a ten-ton truck by an exertion of its "willpower"; similarly, we do not—and should not!—expect an alcoholic or drug addict to "buck up" and resist the overwhelming lure of alcohol or heroin by an exercise of his willpower. The solution to each of these problems is built into the way each is articulated. If the carrying capacity of the bridge is five tons, we must ban vehicles in excess of this weight. If the alcoholic's load limit of liquor is zero, he must not drink. Thus, rehabilitation at Alcoholics Anonymous does not begin until the alcoholic "acknowledges" and publicly declares that he cannot handle liquor—that, in effect, his load limit for alcohol is zero. Our image of the heroin user is similar: we conceive of him as a person whose load limit for heroin is very low or nil, and hence as someone who must, if necessary by external authority or force, be protected from the stress of exposure to it. The prohibition of "dangerous drugs" then follows logically. I hope I need not belabor that this view of the drug abuser or drug addict is wholly metaphorical.

The modern secular view of man assigns an even more distorted role to the tempter. Let us recall that in the old religious view of temptation, the tempter or temptress—for example, the Serpent or Eve in the parable of the Fall—are regarded as responsible agents who commit evil willfully. Their wrongdoing parallels that of the person who yields to temptation, the one in no way affecting the other. The fact that he who tempts commits a wrong does not exonerate him who yields to the temptation. It is not clear who, in theological thought, commits the greater sin—he who tempts or he who yields to temptation. As a rule, the two are not compared. It seems to me, however, that a case might be made for holding the person who succumbs to temptation the greater of the two sinners. I offer this opinion because in the Christian view of the world, temptation is considered to be omnipresent; because it is the duty of the individual to learn to resist it; and, finally, because the source of temptation is often conceived of as non-human or superhuman—that is, diabolical or satanic. It is crucial to this view, moreover, that it promises no hope of eliminating or ridding a person or the world of temptation—once and for all; on the contrary, because it implies that man will always be exposed to temptation, it teaches him to learn to live with it and to try to conquer it.

In the transformation from the religious to the psychiatric view on temptation, this concept of the nature of temptation, and of the tempter or temptress, undergoes a radical change. The responsibility and guilt of the person who succumbs to temptation are abolished, whereas those of the tempter are increased. It is as if the guilt of the fallen tempted were transferred to the successful tempter and then multiplied manyfold. Out of this algebraic transformation of moral burdens arises the "scientific" view of the addict and his supplier: the former is a sick patient who cannot help what he is doing; the latter is a fiendish criminal who could easily help what he is doing. This perspective neatly excludes even the possibility that the addict might be tempted by drugs and the pusher by money, and that each chooses to satisfy rather than to frustrate his particular desire. Nor, of course, is this perspective limited to temptation by drugs or pushers. The same moral mathematics yields the same results for sex: the prostitute, who tempts, is a criminal and is persecuted by the law; her customers, innocent men who succumb to a temptation they could not be expected to resist, are unmolested by the law, or are regarded as "mentally ill" and hence not responsible for their conduct.

There are good reasons, of course, for this remarkable transformation, in the scope of a few centuries, of Western man's most fundamental judgments about success, temptation, and envy. Among these reasons, the two most important ones are the concept of equality and the feeling of envy it engenders. Helmut Schoeck has shown how envy has undergone a transformation identical to that sketched above for temptation: that, in other words, while formerly a person was considered to be evil if he was envious, today he is considered to be evil if he gives others reasons for envying him![14]

It seems to me, however, that envy and covetousness and man's reactions to them are actually only parts of the larger theme of temptation and man's efforts to cope with it. This view is supported by the virtually countless "problems of temptation" in the world; and, more specifically, by the striking similarities between the symbolic meanings and political implications of money and drugs in the two major contemporary ideologies. The socialists and communists, overcome with compassion (genuine or pretended) for the suffering of poor people due to their poverty, and with sympathy for their craving for money, find the incarnation of their enemy in the "capitalists," in "Wall Street," in "private enterprise," and, ultimately, in money itself. Since they condemn what people in fact crave, there remains only one way for them to mitigate their frustration: by eliminating the very thing that people want. Hence the cry to eliminate "profits" and "interest," and to extol "selfless" labor (that is, labor for the State).

The capitalists and therapeutists, overcome with compassion (genuine or pretended) for the suffering of addicted people due to their illness, and with sympathy for their boundless craving for drugs, find the incarnation of their enemy in the "dangerous drug" and the "pusher." Since they too condemn what people in fact crave, there remains only one way for them to mitigate their frustration: by eliminating the very thing that people want. Hence the cry to eliminate "dangerous drugs" and "pushers," and to extol "healthy" living (that is, addiction to drugs mandated by the State).

Because I have categorized the main sources of temptation as knowledge, sex, and power, and because these categories are so broad, they actually encompass a vast range of *doings* and *avoidings* best understood in terms of temptations, but rarely so viewed nowadays. The last category of conduct to which I here want to call attention is that having to do with *defiance*—in particular, with defiance of authority as a means of establishing or safeguarding personal integrity, independence, or a sense of self.

Because man is so profoundly a rule-following being, compliance with or defiance of rules becomes from infancy a part of the human repertoire of action. The baby spitting out food or "refusing" to go to sleep exhibits, and is interpreted by his parents to exhibit, defiance; and he may be dealt with accordingly. All the complicated games that people generate around eating, drinking, urinating, defecating, and sleeping—not to mention sex— often revolve entirely around compliance with or defiance of certain rules governing the use of these body parts. For example, obesity and anorexia nervosa are, in effect, either the results of compliance with commands to overeat or starve (actually or symbolically), or, more often, the results of defiance of rules governing eating. So-called drug abuse and drug addiction often constitute similar patterns of compliance and defiance. It has often been pointed out that many people, especially young persons, use illicit drugs because of peer pressure. Thus, however deviant or defiant such behavior may seem to an outside observer, it is actually, from the subject's point of view, conforming and compliant behavior like any other, except that the rules complied with emanate from a source rejected by accredited authorities. The authority is illegitimate, hence the drugs are "illicit" and "dangerous," and the behavior "sick" and "criminal."

There remains, however, defiance as a motive for using illicit drugs. As I noted, because of man's rule-following nature, every prohibition generates the possibility—and hence the *temptation*—to break the rule and defy the authority who made it and thus enjoy the triumph of successful self-assertion. It is so obvious and so well known that most prohibitions generate massive defiance of them—especially if the prohibited acts supposedly injure only the actor himself, and actually do not injure even him—that I will only record my amazement here about how people can blind themselves to this rule when trying to think about and deal with the "drug problem."

Until masturbation was declared to cause insanity and was prohibited and punished by parents and physicians, it caused no problems. Once these prohibitions were authoritatively articulated and popularly accepted, masturbation became an "epidemic" that swept the civilized world. This epidemic abated, moreover, only when it was replaced by other "epidemics" of temptation-caused "diseases," especially by drug abuse and drug addiction.

I have tried to show that the view which a society and the individuals in it hold concerning the use and avoidance of drugs depends, in very large part, on whether people regard their reasons for doing what they want to do as temptations or as impulses. It matters little whether what people want to do is to kill their unborn babies or elderly relatives, engage in deviant sexual acts, or take drugs that affect their feelings and behavior; whatever the act, we should expect it to be viewed and treated quite differently depending on whether society regards the *actor* as a person yielding to temptation or as a *victim* of an (irresistible) impulse. In the first case, the subject is a culprit or malefactor, and those he injures are his victims; whereas in the second, the subject is not a subject at all, but an object containing, as it were, a bundle of irresistible impulses: hence, he is himself the victim, and those he injures are either ignored and treated as nonexistent or are viewed and treated as the anonymous victims of a natural disaster.

In the former, moral perspective, man is a responsible agent, subject to temptations which he may resist or to which he may yield. In the latter, "scientific" perspective, man is a non-responsible organism, who does not act but displays the consequences of impulses (or drives, instincts, etc.). Obviously, this distinction is not so much theoretical as tactical; it is a distinction whose relevance lies largely in the policies each perspective implies, inspires, and justifies. The imagery of temptation implies the expectation of self-control; whereas the imagery of impulse implies a need for external controls.

If this general perspective on behavior regulation is valid, we would expect not only that certain social problems—in particular, drug abuse and drug addiction, which remain our main concerns here—would be viewed very differently in societies which are imbued, respectively, with a religious or scientific outlook, but also that, for the reasons discussed earlier, dangerous drugs would not be much of a problem in the former but would assume gigantic proportions in the latter. And so indeed it is. In Ireland and Israel, the problem of drug abuse is insignificant; whereas in Sweden and the United States—and in other countries where drug use is viewed in terms of impulse instead of temptation, in terms of psychiatry instead of religion, in terms of sickness instead of sin—the problem is immense and intractable. I would thus venture to suggest that, to the extent to which the people in these latter countries continue to expect personal conduct to be regulated less and less by the person himself and more and more by the medical profession acting through the state, the problem of drug abuse will grow rather than diminish.

All that I have said so far points to this conclusion: that the imagery and vocabulary of both "temptation" and "impulse" is tactical rather than descriptive. We speak of temptations when we want and expect people to control themselves; and of impulses when we want and expect them to be controlled by other people.

Because social existence is inconceivable without controls on human behavior; and because human behavior can be controlled in two ways, and two ways only—by internal or external controls, that is, by self-control or by external coercion—it is easy to see why both of the foregoing images and vocabularies have always been with us, and probably always will be. When our religions were theological rather than therapeutic, we emphasized temptation and self-control more than we do now. But it would be a mistake to glamorize the Judeo-Christian religions for emphasizing the value of self-control more than they really did; in actuality, they always relied heavily on external controls exercised by religious authorities; they also assigned controls to metaphorical and mythological entities, like demons and the devil, which, though "inside" the person, were conceived as distinct and separate from him. The concept of "schizophrenia"—of a split personality or a divided self—is thus inherent in the Judeo-Christian view of man: in its original, pristine form, this concept was articulated as "possession"—that is, as man struggling against the devil that has "possessed" him; then the concept became articulated as madness or insanity—that is, as man struggling against irresistible impulses that "control" him; finally it became articulated as "schizophrenia"—that is, as different parts of the "personality" locked in a struggle with each other.

If we want to understand our "drug problem," or almost any other psychiatric problem, we must not use terms like "temptation," "impulse," "drug abuse," or "schizophrenia," because each prejudges the phenomena we are trying to understand and describe. Instead, we must speak simply in terms of behavior and its control. "Temptation" and "impulse" will then be seen as two types of behavior controls: the former is an attempt to induce or reward a certain kind of behavior in someone else, which the person describing the behavior believes should not be rewarded, or should not be rewarded in the way the tempter proposes; and the latter is an attempt to induce or reward a certain kind of behavior in oneself, which, again, the person describing it believes should not be rewarded or not in the way proposed. "Schizophrenia" will then be seen as the name of a particular consequence of a series of antecedent behavior controls of which the person describing it disapproves.

To deal with the practical—intellectual, moral, and political—problems that behavior controls present to us, we must discard all of these images and vocabularies; and must approach our subject more simply and directly. Let me indicate briefly what seems to me a promising approach in thinking about this subject.

First, a person may try to eliminate—destroy, as it were—a temptation. This is effective only if a person imposes a prohibition on himself, or subjects himself willingly to a prohibition imposed on him by the authorities. Monks withdrawing into the desert protected themselves from the temptation of women; Luther chose marriage. The point to remember here is that the very process of forbidding something calls it to mind; hence the familiar adage about forbidden fruit tasting sweeter. The Original Sin is an instance of an attempt, on God's part, to forbid a particular act, the prohibition serving only to make it into an "irresistible" temptation to which man and woman succumb.

Second, a person (or group) may warn others of the consequences of certain acts. The sign "Danger: High Voltage!" is this sort of communication. Of course, even a warning may serve as a temptation, for example to those who might want to commit suicide by electrocuting themselves, or who might want to sabotage a high-voltage line.

Third, a person (or group) may try to deal with what might be a temptation for others by ignoring it, mentioning it as little as possible, perhaps even by not giving it a name. This is an exceedingly important—and nowadays widely used but rarely discussed—method of behavior control in all modern societies. It plays an especially prominent role in totalitarian politics and history: if dissidents disappear without a trace, or if Trotsky is not mentioned in Soviet history texts, then Russians will have scant temptation to think about them or to revere them.

These considerations make it abundantly clear why our present war on drug abuse encourages precisely the sort of behavior which its stupid or sadistic supporters claim they want to discourage. Indeed, this is so obvious that it hardly deserves serious discussion. What is much less obvious is why these kinds of self-defeating, "counterproductive" social policies are so popular, especially in the United States. No doubt one of the reasons why such policies might be attractive to modern people everywhere, and perhaps especially in the United States, is because they allow them to be childish and dependent on authorities, while continuing to regard themselves as remaining "politically independent." When Americans depend for drug controls not on themselves, but on anti-drug laws (that is, they cast their votes for laws that take drugs away from themselves); when they depend for alcohol controls not on themselves, but on Alcoholics Anonymous; when they depend for weight control not on themselves, but on Weight Watchers; and when, in general, they depend for the control of every vicissitude of human existence not on themselves, but on doctors and diagnoses and drugs—they can nevertheless still feel "free" and "politically independent," because they are not visibly tyrannized by a Hitler or Stalin!

Man's ability to deceive others is exceeded only by his ability to deceive himself. So-called addictive drugs often help a person to deceive himself; but they also help him to escape from the authorities who deceive him. This is why drug controls get so easily out of hand. The authorities try to monopolize all methods of interpersonal control, including drugs and deception about drugs: They declare war on all those drugs that the people themselves want to take; and they insist on deciding what drugs to give to the people, or even to force upon them.

12. THE CONTROL OF CONDUCT: AUTHORITY VERSUS AUTONOMY

There is only one political sin: independence; and only one political virtue: obedience. To put it differently, there is only one offense against authority: self-control; and only one obeisance to it: submission to control by authority.

Why is self-control, autonomy, such a threat to authority? Because the person who controls himself, who is his own master, has no need for an authority to be his master. This, then, renders authority unemployed. What is he to do if he cannot control others? To be sure, he could mind his own business. But this is a fatuous answer, for those who are satisfied to mind their own business do not aspire to become authorities. In short, authority needs subjects, persons not in command of themselves—just as parents need children and physicians need patients.

Autonomy is the death knell of authority, and authority knows it: hence the ceaseless warfare of authority against the exercise, both real and symbolic, of autonomy—that is, against suicide, against masturbation, against self-medication, against the proper use of language itself![1]

The parable of the Fall illustrates this fight to the death between control and self-control. Did Eve, tempted by the Serpent, seduce Adam, who then lost control of himself and succumbed to evil? Or did Adam, facing a choice between obedience to the authority of God and his own destiny, choose self-control?

How, then, shall we view the situation of the so-called drug abuser or drug addict? As a stupid, sick, and helpless child, who, tempted by pushers, peers, and the pleasures of drugs, succumbs to the lure and loses control of himself? Or as a person in control of himself, who, like Adam, chooses the forbidden fruit as the elemental and elementary way of pitting himself against authority?

There is no empirical or scientific way of choosing between these two answers, of deciding which is right and which is wrong. The questions frame two different moral perspectives, and the answers define two different moral strategies: if we side with authority and wish to repress the individual, we shall treat him *as if* he were helpless, the innocent victim of overwhelming temptation; and we shall then "protect" him from further temptation by treating him as a child, slave, or madman. If we side with the individual and wish to refute the legitimacy and reject the power of authority to infantilize him, we shall treat him *as if* he were in command of himself, the executor of responsible decisions; and we shall then demand that he respect others as he respects himself by treating him as an adult, a free individual, or a "rational" person.

Either of these positions makes sense. What makes less sense—what is confusing in principle and chaotic practice—is to treat people as adults *and* children, as free and unfree, as sane and insane.

Nevertheless, this is just what social authorities throughout history have done: in ancient Greece, in medieval Europe, in the contemporary world, we find various mixtures in the attitudes of the authorities toward the people; in some societies, the individual is treated as more free than unfree, and we call these societies "free"; in others, he is treated as more determined than self-determining, and we call these societies "totalitarian." In none is the individual treated as completely free. Perhaps this would be impossible: many persons insist that no society could survive on such a premise consistently carried through. Perhaps this is something that lies in the future of mankind. In any case, we should take satisfaction in the evident impossibility of the opposite situation: no society has ever treated the individual, nor perhaps could it treat him, as completely determined. The apparent freedom of the authority, controlling both himself and subject, provides an irresistible model: if God can control, if pope and prince can control, if politician and psychiatrist can control—then perhaps the person can also control, at least himself.

The conflicts between those who have power and those who want to take it away from them fall into three distinct categories. In moral, political, and social affairs (and I of course include psychiatric affairs among these), these categories must be clearly distinguished; if we do not distinguish among them we are likely to mistake opposition to absolute or arbitrary power with what may, actually, be an attempt to gain such power for oneself or for the groups or leaders one admires.

First, there are those who want to take power away from the oppressor and give it to the oppressed, as a class—as exemplified by Marx, Lenin, and the Communists. Revealingly, they dream of the "dictatorship" of the proletariat or some other group.

Second, there are those who want to take power away from the oppressor and give it to themselves as the protectors of the oppressed—as exemplified by Robespierre in politics; Rush in medicine; and by their liberal, radical, and medical followers. Revealingly, they dream of the incorruptibly honest or incontrovertibly sane ruler leading his happy or healthy flock.

And third, there are those who want to take power away from the oppressor and give it to the oppressed as individuals, for each to do with as he pleases, but hopefully for his own self-control—as exemplified by Mill, von Mises, the free-market economists, and their libertarian followers. Revealingly, they dream of people so self-governing that their need for and tolerance of rulers is minimal or nil.

While countless men say they love liberty, clearly only those who, by virtue of their actions, fall into the third category, mean it.[2] The others merely want to replace a hated oppressor by a loved one—having usually themselves in mind for the job.

As we have seen, psychiatrists (and some other physicians, notably public health administrators) have traditionally opted for "reforms" of the second type; that is, their opposition to existing powers, ecclesiastic or secular, has had as its conscious and avowed aim the paternalistic care of the citizen-patient, and not the freedom of the autonomous individual. Hence, medical methods of social control tended not only to replace religious methods, but sometimes to exceed them in stringency and severity. In short, the usual response of medical authority to the controls exercised by non-medical authority has been to try to take over and then escalate the controls, rather than to endorse the principle and promote the practice of removing the controls by which the oppressed are victimized.

As a result, until recently, most psychiatrists, psychologists, and other behavioral scientists had nothing but praise for the "behavioral controls" of medicine and psychiatry. We are now beginning to witness, however, a seeming backlash against this position, many behavioral scientists jumping on what they evidently consider to be the next "correct" and "liberal" position, namely, a criticism of behavioral controls. But since most of these "scientists" remain as hostile to individual freedom and responsibility, to choice and dignity, as they have always been, their criticism conforms to the pattern I have described above: they demand more "controls"—that is, professional and governmental controls —over "behavior controls." This is like first urging a person to drive over icy roads at breakneck speed to get over them as fast as possible, and then, when his car goes into a skid, advising him to apply his brakes. Whether because they are stupid or wicked or both, such persons invariably recommend fewer controls where more are needed, for example in relation to punishing offenders— and more controls where fewer are needed, for example in relation to contracts between consenting adults. Truly, the supporters of the Therapeutic State are countless and tireless—now proposing more therapeutic controls in the name of "controlling behavior controls."[3]

Clearly, the seeds of this fundamental human propensity—to react to the loss of control, or to the threat of such loss, with an intensification of control, thus generating a spiraling symbiosis of escalating controls and counter-controls—have fallen on fertile soil in contemporary medicine and psychiatry and have yielded a luxuriant harvest of "therapeutic" coercions. The alcoholic and Alcoholics Anonymous, the glutton and Weight Watchers, the drug abuser and the drug-abuseologist—each is an image at war with its mirror image, each creating and defining, dignifying and defaming the other, and each trying to negate his own reflection, which he can accomplish only by negating himself.

There is only one way to split apart and unlock such pairings, to resolve such dilemmas—namely, by trying to control the other less, not more; and by replacing control of the other with self-control.

The person who uses drugs—legal or illegal drugs, with or without a physician's prescription—may be submitting to authority, may be revolting against it, or may be exercising his own power of making a free decision. It is quite impossible to know—without knowing a great deal about such a person, his family and friends, and his whole cultural setting—just what such an individual is doing and why. But it is quite possible, indeed it is easy, to know what those persons who try to repress certain kinds of drug uses and drug users are doing and why.

As the war against heresy was in reality a war for "true" faith, so the war against drug abuse is in reality a war for "faithful" drug use: concealed behind the war against marijuana and heroin is the war for tobacco and alcohol; and, more generally, concealed behind the war against the use of politically and medically disapproved drugs, is the war for the use of politically and medically approved drugs.

Let us recall, again, one of the principles implicit in the psychiatric perspective on man, and some of the practices that follow from it: the madman is a person lacking adequate internal controls over his behavior hence, he requires—for his own protection as well as for the protection of society—external restraints upon it. This, then, justifies the incarceration of "mental patients" in "mental hospitals"—and much else besides.

The drug abuser is a person lacking adequate internal controls over his drug use; hence, he requires—for his own protection as well as for the protection of society—external restraints upon it. This, then, justifies the prohibition of "dangerous drugs," the incarceration and involuntary treatment of "addicts," the eradication of "pushers"—and much else besides.

Confronted with the phenomena of "drug abuse" and "drug addiction," how else could psychiatry and a society imbued with it have reacted? They could respond only as they did—namely, by defining the moderate use of legal drugs as the result of the sane control of resistible impulses; and by defining the immoderate use of any drug, and any use of illegal drugs, as the insane surrender to irresistible impulses. Hence the circular psychiatric definitions of drug habits, such as the claim that illicit drug use (for example, smoking marijuana) causes mental illness and also constitutes a symptom of it; and the seemingly contradictory claim that the wholly similar use of licit drugs (for example, smoking tobacco) is neither a cause nor a symptom of mental illness.

Formerly, opium was a panacea; now it is the cause and symptom of countless maladies, medical and social, the world over. Formerly masturbation was the cause and symptom of mental illness; now it is the cure for social inhibition and the practice ground for training in heterosexual athleticism. It is clear, then, that if we want to understand and accept drug-taking behavior, we must take a larger view of the so-called drug problem. (Of course, if we want to persecute "pushers" and "treat addicts," then information inconvenient to our doing these things will only get in our way. Drug-abuseologists can no more be "educated" out of their coercive tactics than can drug addicts.)

What does this larger view show us? How can it help us? It shows us that our present attitudes toward the whole subject of drug use, drug abuse, and drug control are nothing but the reflections, in the mirror of "social reality," of our own expectations toward drugs and toward those who use them; and that our ideas about and interventions in drug-taking behavior have only the most tenuous connection with the actual pharmacological properties of "dangerous drugs." The "danger" of masturbation disappeared when we ceased to believe in it: we then ceased to attribute danger to the practice and to its practitioners; and ceased to call it "self-abuse."

Of course, some people still behave in disagreeable and even dangerous ways, but we no longer attribute their behavior to masturbation or self-abuse: we now attribute their behavior to self-medication or drug abuse. We thus play a game of musical chairs with medical alibis for human desire, determination, and depravity. Though this sort of intolerance is easy, it is also expensive: it seems clear that only in accepting human beings for what they are can we accept the chemical substances they use for what they are. In short, only insofar as we are able and willing to accept men, women, and children as neither angels nor devils, but as persons with certain inalienable rights and irrepudiable duties, shall we be able and willing to accept heroin, cocaine, and marijuana as neither panaceas nor panapathogens, but as drugs with certain chemical properties and ceremonial possibilities.

Appendix
A Synoptic History of the Promotion and Prohibition of Drugs

In the following synoptic history of the promotion and prohibition of drugs, I try to provide, in relatively compact form, a large amount of information on one of man's basic passions—using and avoiding drugs. Ignorance of these facts, or their deliberate neglect, renders virtually all contemporary debates, discussions, commission reports, and legislative proposals concerning the so-called drug problem both foolish and useless. I hope that this material will not only inform and instruct the reader, but also shame and shock him into a fuller realization of the horrifying intemperance of both those who zealously promote and those who zealously prohibit drugs.

c. 5000 B.C.   The Sumerians use opium, suggested by the fact that they have an ideogram for it which has been translated as HUL, meaning "joy" or "rejoicing."[1]

c. 3500 B.C.   Earliest historical record of the production of alcohol: the description of a brewery in an Egyptian papyrus.[2]

c. 3000 B.C.   Approximate date of the supposed origin of the use of tea in China.

c. 2500 B.C.   Earliest historical evidence of the eating of poppy seeds among the Lake Dwellers of Switzerland.[3]

c. 2000 B.C.   Earliest record of prohibitionist teaching, by an Egyptian priest, who writes to his pupil: "I, thy superior, forbid thee to go to the taverns. Thou art degraded like the beasts."[4]

c. 350 B.C.   Proverbs, 31:6–7: "Give strong drink to him who is perishing, and wine to those in bitter distress; let them drink and forget their poverty, and remember their misery no more."

c. 300 B.C.   Theophrastus (371–287 B.C.), Greek naturalist and philosopher, records what has remained as the earliest undisputed reference to the use of the poppy juice.

c. 250 B.C.   Psalms, 104:14–15: "Thou dost cause grass to grow for the cattle, and plants for man to cultivate, that he may bring forth food from the earth, and wine to gladden the heart of man."

350 A.D.   Earliest written mention of tea, in a Chinese dictionary.

4th century   St. John Chrysostom (345–407), Bishop of Constantinople: "I hear man cry, 'Would there be no wine! O folly! O madness!' Is it wine that causes this abuse? No. For if you say, 'Would there be no wine!' because of drunkenness, then you must say, going on by degrees, 'Would there were no night!' because of the thieves, 'Would there were no light!' because of the informers, and 'Would there were no women!' because of adultery."[5]

c. 450   Babylonian Talmud: "Wine is at the head of all medicines; where wine is lacking, drugs are necessary."[6]

c. 1000   Opium is widely used in China and the Far East.[7]

1229   The ecclesiastic authorities of Toulouse declare: "We also forbid the laity to possess any of the books of the Old or New Testament . . . that any should have these books translated into the vulgar tongue we strictly forbid."[8]

1382   John Wycliffe completes his translation of the Bible into English.

1493   The use of tobacco is introduced into Europe by Columbus and his crew returning from America.

c. 1500   According to J. D. Rolleston, a British medical

historian, a medieval Russian cure for drunkenness consisted "in taking a piece of pork, putting it secretly into a Jew's bed for nine days, and then giving it to the drunkard in a pulverized form, who will turn away from drinking as a Jew would from pork."[9]

c. 1525   Paracelsus (1490–1541) introduces laudanum, or tincture of opium, into the practice of medicine.

1526   Six thousand copies of Tyndale's English Bible are printed at Worms and smuggled into England.[10]

1529   Charles V (1500–58), Holy Roman Emperor and ruler of the Netherlands, decrees that the "reading, purchasing, or possessing any proscribed books, or any New Testaments prohibited by the theologians of Louvain" are crimes, the punishments for which are that "the men be beheaded, the women buried alive, and the relapsed burned."[11]

1536   William Tyndale, translator of the New Testament and the Pentateuch, is burned at the stake as a heretic, at Vilvorde Castle, near Brussels.

1559   Valdes' Spanish Index, decreeing the prohibition of all religious literature in the language of the people, is published. The penalty for possessing prohibited books is death.[12]

1600   Shakespeare: "Falstaff. . . . If I had a thousand sons, the / first human principle I would teach them should / be, to foreswear thin potations and to addict themselves to sack." ("Sack," a term now obsolete, meant strong sweet wine, for example a sherry.)[13]

17th century   The prince of the petty state of Waldeck pays ten thalers to anyone who denounces a coffee drinker.[14]

17th century   In Russia, Czar Michael Federovitch executes anyone on whom tobacco is found. "Czar Alexei Mikhailovitch rules that anyone caught with tobacco should be tortured until he gave up the name of the supplier."[15]

1601   The Spanish Dominican Alonso Giroi demands the complete prohibition of all religious books in the people's language.[16]

1613   John Rolfe, the husband of the Indian princess Pocahontas, sends the first shipment of Virginia tobacco from Jamestown to England.

c. 1650   The use of tobacco is prohibited in Bavaria, Saxony, and Zürich, but the prohibitions are ineffective. Sultan Murad IV of the Ottoman Empire decrees the death penalty for smoking tobacco: "Wherever the Sultan went on his travels or on a military expedition his halting-places were always distinguished by a terrible increase in the number of executions. Even on the battlefield he was fond of surprising men in the act of smoking, when he would punish them by beheading, hanging, quartering or crushing their hands and feet. . . . Nevertheless, in spite of all the horrors of this persecution . . . the passion for smoking still persisted."[17]

1680   Thomas Sydenham (1624–80): "Among the remedies which it has pleased the Almighty God to give to man to relieve his sufferings, none is so universal and so efficacious as opium."[18]

1690   The "Act for the Encouraging of the Distillation of Brandy and Spirits from Corn" is enacted in England.[19]

1691   In Luneberg, Germany, the penalty for smoking (tobacco) is death.[20]

1717   Liquor licenses in Middlesex (England) are granted only to those who "would take oaths of allegiance and of belief in the King's supremacy over the Church."[21]

1736   The Gin Act (England) is enacted with the avowed objects of making spirits "come so dear to the consumer that the poor will not be able to launch out into an excessive use of them." This effort results in general lawbreaking and fails to halt the steady rise in the consumption of even legally produced and sold liquor.[22]

1745   The magistrates of one London division demand that "publicans and wine-merchants should swear that they anathematized the doctrine of Transubstantiation."[23]

1762   Thomas Dover, an English physician, introduces his prescription for a "diaphoretic powder," which he recommends mainly for the treatment of gout. Soon named "Dover's powder," this compound becomes one of the most widely used opium preparations during the next 150 years.

1770   Women in New England organize boycotts against tea imported from Britain; some of these associations call themselves "Daughters of Liberty," their members pledging themselves not to drink tea until after the Revenue Act is repealed. They also popularize various tea substitutes—such as brews of raspberry, sage, and birch leaves—the most popular of which, made from the four-leaved loosestrife, is called "Liberty Tea."[24]

1773   To protest the tax on tea, a band of Bostonians, dressed as Mohawk Indians, boards three British ships in Boston Harbor and throws overboard 342 chests of tea (December 16, 1773). This episode leads to the passage of the Coercive Acts (1774) by the British Parliament, which, in turn, leads to the assembly of the First Continental Congress (September 5, 1774) and to the War of Independence and the birth of the United States as a nation.

1785   Benjamin Rush publishes his *Inquiry into the Ef-*

fects of *Ardent Spirits on the Human Body and Mind;* in it, he calls the intemperate use of distilled spirits a "disease," and estimates the annual rate of death due to alcoholism in the United States as "not less than 4,000 people" in a population then of less than 6 million.[25]

1789   The first American temperance society is formed in Litchfield, Connecticut.[26]

1790   Benjamin Rush persuades his associates at the Philadelphia College of Physicians to send an appeal to Congress to "impose such heavy duties upon all distilled spirits as shall be effective to restrain their intemperate use in the country."[27]

1792   The first prohibitory laws against opium in China are promulgated. The punishment decreed for keepers of opium shops is strangulation.

1794   The Whisky Rebellion, a protest by farmers in western Pennsylvania against a federal tax on liquor, breaks out and is put down by overwhelming force sent into the area by George Washington.

1797   Samuel Taylor Coleridge writes "Kubla Khan" while under the influence of opium.

1800   Napoleon's army, returning from Egypt, introduces cannabis (hashish, marijuana) into France. Avant-garde artists and writers in Paris develop their own cannabis ritual, leading, in 1844, to the establishment of *Le Club des Haschischins.*[28]

1801   On Jefferson's recommendation, the federal duty on liquor is abolished.[29]

1804   Thomas Trotter, an Edinburgh physician, publishes *An Essay, Medical, Philosophical, and Chemical, on Drunkenness and Its Effects on the Human Body:* "In medical language, I consider drunkenness, strictly speaking, to be a disease, produced by a remote cause, and giving birth to actions and movements in the living body that disorder the functions of health. . . . The habit of drunkenness is a disease of the mind."[30]

1805   Friedrich Wilhelm Adam Sertürner, a German chemist, isolates and describes morphine.

1822   Thomas De Quincey's *Confessions of an English Opium Eater* is published. He notes that the opium habit, like any other habit, must be learned: "Making allowance for constitutional differences, I should say that *in less than 120 days* no habit of opium-eating could be formed strong enough to call for any extraordinary self-conquest in renouncing it, and even suddenly renouncing it. On Saturday you are an opium-eater, on Sunday no longer such."[31]

1826   The American Society for the Promotion of Temperance is founded in Boston. By 1833, there are 6,000 local Temperance societies, with more than one million members.

1839–42   The First Opium War. The British force upon China the trade in opium, a trade the Chinese had declared illegal.[32]

1840   Benjamin Parsons, an English clergyman, declares: ". . . alcohol stands preeminent as a destroyer. . . . I never knew a person become insane who was not in the habit of taking a portion of alcohol every day." Parsons lists forty-two distinct diseases caused by alcohol, among them inflammation of the brain, scrofula, mania, dropsy, nephritis, and gout.[33]

1841   Dr. Jacques Joseph Moreau uses hashish in treating mental patients at the Bicêtre.[34]

1842   Abraham Lincoln: "In my judgment, such of us as have never fallen victims, have been spared more from the absence of appetite, than from any mental or moral superiority over those who have. Indeed, I believe, if we take habitual drunkards as a class, their heads and their hearts will bear an advantageous comparison with those of any other class."[35]

1844   Cocaine is isolated in pure form.

1845   A law prohibiting the public sale of liquor is enacted in New York State. It is repealed in 1847.

1847   The American Medical Association is founded.

1852   Susan B. Anthony establishes the Woman's State Temperance Society of New York, the first such society formed by and for women. Many of the early feminists, such as Elizabeth Cady Stanton, Lucretia Mott, and Abby Kelly, are also ardent prohibitionists.[36]

1852   The American Pharmaceutical Association is founded. The Association's 1856 Constitution lists one of its goals as: "To as much as possible restrict the dispensing and sale of medicines to regularly educated druggists and apothecaries."[37]

1856   The Second Opium War. The British, with help from the French, extend their powers to distribute opium in China.

1862   Internal Revenue Act enacted imposing a license fee of twenty dollars on retail liquor dealers, and a tax of one dollar a barrel on beer and twenty cents a gallon on spirits.[38]

1864   Adolf von Baeyer, a twenty-nine-year-old assistant of Friedrich August Kekule (the discoverer of the molecular structure of benzene) in Ghent, synthesizes barbituric acid, the first barbiturate.

1868   Dr. George Wood, professor of the theory and practice of medicine at the University of Pennsylvania, president of the American Philosophical Society, and the author of a leading American text, *Treatise on Therapeutics,* describes the pharmacological effect of opium as follows: "A sensation of fullness is felt in the head, soon followed by a universal feeling of delicious ease and comfort, with an elevation and expansion of the whole moral and intellectual nature, which is, I think, the most characteristic of its effects . . . the intellectual and imaginative faculties are raised to the highest point compatible with individual capacity. . . . It seems to make the individual, for the time, a better and greater man. . . . The hallucinations, the delirious imaginations of alcoholic intoxication, are, in general, quite wanting. Along with this emotional and intellectual elevation, there is also increased muscular energy; and the capacity to act, and to bear fatigue, is greatly augmented."[39]

1869   The Prohibition Party is formed. Gerrit Smith, twice Abolitionist candidate for President, an associate of John Brown, and a crusading prohibitionist, declares: "Our involuntary slaves are set free, but our millions of voluntary slaves still clang their chains. The lot of the literal slave, of him whom others have enslaved, is indeed a hard one; nevertheless, it is a paradise compared with the lot of him who enslaves himself—especially of him who has enslaved himself to alcohol."[40]

1874   The Woman's Christian Temperance Union is founded in Cleveland. In 1883, Frances Willard, a leader of the W.C.T.U., forms the World's Woman's Christian Temperance Union.

1882   The first law in the United States, and in the world, making "temperance education" a part of the required course in public schools is enacted. In 1886, Congress makes such education mandatory in the District of Columbia, and in territorial, military, and naval schools. By 1900, all the states have similar laws.[41]

1882   The Personal Liberty League of the United States is founded to oppose the increasing momentum of movements for compulsory abstinence from alcohol.[42]

1883   Dr. Theodor Aschenbrandt, a German army physician, secures a supply of pure cocaine from the pharmaceutical firm of Merck, issues it to Bavarian soldiers during their maneuvers, and reports on the beneficial effects of the drug in increasing the soldiers' ability to endure fatigue.[43]

1884   Sigmund Freud treats his depression with cocaine, and reports feeling "exhilaration and lasting euphoria, which in no way differs from the normal euphoria of the healthy person. . . . You perceive an increase in self-control and possess more vitality and capacity for work. . . . In other words, you are simply more normal, and it is soon hard to believe that you are under the influence of any drug."[44]

1884   Laws are enacted to make anti-alcohol teaching compulsory in public schools in New York State. The following year similar laws are passed in Pennsylvania, with other states soon following suit.

1885   The Report of the Royal Commission on Opium concludes that opium is more like the Westerner's liquor than a substance to be feared and abhorred.[45]

1889   The Johns Hopkins Hospital, in Baltimore, Maryland, is opened. One of its world-famous founders, Dr. William Stewart Halsted, is a morphine addict. He continues to use morphine in large doses throughout a phenomenally successful surgical career lasting until his death in 1922.

1894   The Report of the Indian Hemp Drug Commission, running to over three thousand pages in seven volumes, is published. This inquiry, commissioned by the British government, concludes: "There is no evidence of any weight regarding the mental and moral injuries from the moderate use of these drugs. . . . Moderation does not lead to excess in hemp any more than it does in alcohol. Regular, moderate use of ganja or bhang produces the same effects as moderate and regular doses of whiskey." The Commission's proposal to tax bhang is never put into effect, in part, perhaps, because one of the Commissioners, an Indian, cautions that Moslem law and Hindu custom forbid "taxing anything that gives pleasure to the poor."[46]

1894   Norman Kerr, an English physician and president of the British Society for the Study of Inebriety, declares: "Drunkenness has generally been regarded as . . . a sin, a vice, or a crime. . . . [But] there is now a consensus of intelligent opinion that habitual and periodic drunkenness is often either a symptom or a sequel of disease . . . a functional neurotic disease, and may be considered as one of a group of nervous affections. . . . The victim can no more resist [alcohol] than a man with ague can resist shivering."[47]

1898   Diacetylmorphine (heroin) is synthesized in Germany. It is widely lauded as a "safe preparation free from addiction-forming properties."[48]

1900   In an address to the Ecumenical Missionary Conference, Rev. Wilbur F. Crafts declares: "No Christian celebration of the completion of nineteen Christian centuries has yet been arranged. Could there be a fitter one than the general adoption, by separate and joint action of the great nations of the world, of the new policy of civilization, in which Great Britain is leading, the policy of prohibition for native races, in the interest of commerce as well as conscience, since the liquor traffic among child races, even more manifestly than in civilized lands, injures all other trades by producing poverty, disease, and death. Our object, more profoundly viewed, is to create a more favorable environment for the child races that civilized nations are essaying to civilize and Christianize."[49]

1900   James R. L. Daly, writing in the *Boston Medical and Surgical Journal,* declares: "It [heroin] possesses many advantages over morphine. . . . It is not hypnotic; there is no danger of acquiring the habit . . ."[50]

1901   The Senate adopts a resolution, introduced by Henry Cabot Lodge, to forbid the sale by American traders of opium and alcohol "to aboriginal tribes and uncivilized races." These provisions are later extended to include "uncivilized elements in America itself and in its territories, such as Indians, Alaskans, the inhabitants of Hawaii, railroad workers, and immigrants at ports of entry."[51]

1901   In Colorado, a bill is introduced, but is defeated, making not only morphine and cocaine but also "malt, vinous and spiritous liquors" available only on a physician's prescription.[52]

1902   The Committee on the Acquirement of the Drug Habit of the American Pharmaceutical Association declares: "If the Chinaman cannot get along without his 'dope,' we can get along without him."[53]

1902   George E. Petey, writing in the *Alabama Medical Journal,* observes: "Many articles have appeared in the medical literature during the last two years lauding this new agent. . . . When we consider the fact that heroin is a morphine derivative . . . it does not seem reasonable that such a claim could be well founded. It is strange that such a claim should mislead anyone or that there should be found among the members of our profession those who would reiterate and accentuate it without first subjecting it to the most critical tests, but such is the fact."[54]

1903   The composition of Coca-Cola is changed, caffeine replacing the cocaine it contained until this time.[55]

1904   Charles Lyman, president of the International Reform Bureau, petitions the President of the United States "to induce Great Britain to release China from the enforced opium traffic. . . . We need not recall in detail that China prohibited the sale of opium, except as a medicine, until the sale was forced upon that country by Great Britain in the opium war of 1840."[56]

1905   Senator Henry W. Blair, in a letter to Rev. Wilbur F. Crafts, Superintendent of the International Reform Bureau: "The temperance movement must include all poisonous substances which create or excite unnatural appetite, and international prohibition is the goal."[57]

1906   The first Pure Food and Drug Act becomes law; until its enactment, it was possible to buy, in stores or by mail order, medicines containing morphine, cocaine, or heroin, and without their being so labeled.

1906   *Squibb's Materia Medica* lists heroin as "a remedy of much value . . . it is also used as a mild anodyne and as a substitute for morphine in combating the morphine habit."[58]

1909   The United States prohibits the importation of smoking opium.[59]

1910   Dr. Hamilton Wright, considered by some the father of U.S. anti-narcotics laws, reports that American contractors give cocaine to their Negro employees to get more work out of them.[60]

1912   A writer in *Century* magazine proclaims: "The

relation of tobacco, especially in the form of cigarettes, and alcohol and opium is a very close one. . . . Morphine is the legitimate consequence of alcohol, and alcohol is the legitimate consequence of tobacco. Cigarettes, drink, opium, is the logical and regular series." And a physician warns: "[There is] no energy more destructive of soul, mind, and body, or more subversive of good morals, than the cigarette. The fight against the cigarette is a fight for civilization."[61]

1912   The first international Opium Convention meets at The Hague, and recommends various measures for the international control of the trade in opium. Subsequent Opium Conventions are held in 1913 and 1914.

1912   Phenobarbital is introduced into therapeutics under the trade name of Luminal.

1913   The Sixteenth Amendment, creating the legal authority for a federal income tax, is enacted. Between 1870 and 1915, the tax on liquor provides from one-half to two-thirds of the whole of the internal revenue of the United States, amounting, after the turn of the century, to about $200 million annually. The Sixteenth Amendment thus makes possible, just seven years later, the Eighteenth Amendment.

1914   The Harrison Narcotic Act is enacted, controlling the sale of opium and opium derivatives.

1914   Congressman Richard P. Hobson of Alabama, urging a prohibition amendment to the Constitution, asserts: "Liquor will actually make a brute out of a negro, causing him to commit unnatural crimes. The effect is the same on the white man, though the white man being further evolved it takes longer time to reduce him to the same level." Negro leaders join the crusade against alcohol.[62]

1916   The *Pharmacopoeia of the United States* drops whiskey and brandy from its list of drugs. Four years later, American physicians begin prescribing these "drugs" in quantities never before prescribed by doctors.

1917   The president of the American Medical Association endorses national prohibition. The House of Delegates of the Association passes a resolution stating: "Resolved, The American Medical Association opposes the use of alcohol as a beverage; and be it further Resolved, That the use of alcohol as a therapeutic agent should be discouraged." By 1928, physicians make an estimated $40,000,000 annually by writing prescriptions for whiskey.[63]

1917   The American Medical Association passes a resolution declaring that "sexual continence is compatible with health and is the best prevention of venereal infections," and that one of the methods for controlling syphilis is by controlling alcohol. Secretary of the Navy Josephus Daniels prohibits the practice of distributing contraceptives to sailors bound on shore leave, and Congress passes laws setting up "dry and decent zones" around military camps. "Many barkeepers are fined for selling liquor to men in uniform. Only at Coney Island could soldiers and sailors change into the grateful anonymity of bathing suits and drink without molestation from patriotic passers-by."[64]

1918   The Anti-Saloon League calls the "liquor traffic" "un-American, pro-German, crime-producing, food-wasting, youth-corrupting, home-wrecking, [and] treasonable."[65]

1919   The Eighteenth (Prohibition) Amendment is added to the U. S. Constitution. It is repealed in 1933.

1920   The U. S. Department of Agriculture publishes

a pamphlet urging Americans to grow cannabis (marijuana) as a profitable undertaking.[66]

1920–33
The use of alcohol is prohibited in the United States. In 1932 alone, approximately 45,000 persons receive jail sentences for alcohol offenses. During the first eleven years of the Volstead Act, 17,972 persons are appointed to the Prohibition Bureau, 11,982 are terminated "without prejudice," and 1,604 are dismissed for bribery, extortion, theft, falsification of records, conspiracy, forgery, and perjury.[67]

1921
The U. S. Treasury Department issues regulations outlining the treatment of addiction permitted under the Harrison Act. In Syracuse, New York, the narcotics clinic doctors report curing 90 per cent of their addicts.[68]

1921
Thomas S. Blair, M.D., chief of the Bureau of Drug Control of the Pennsylvania Department of Health, publishes a paper in the *Journal of the American Medical Association* in which he characterizes the Indian peyote religion a "habit indulgence in certain cactaceous plants," calls the belief system a "superstition" and those who sell peyote "dope vendors," and urges the passage of a bill in Congress that would prohibit the use of peyote among the Indian tribes of the Southwest. He concludes with this revealing plea for abolition: "The great difficulty in suppressing this habit among the Indians arises from the fact that the commercial interests involved in the peyote traffic are strongly entrenched, and they exploit the Indian. . . . Added to this is the superstition of the Indian who believes in the Peyote Church. As soon as an effort is made to suppress peyote, the cry is raised that it is unconstitutional to do so and is an invasion of religious liberty. Sup-

pose the negroes of the South had a Cocaine Church!"[69]

1921   Cigarettes are illegal in fourteen states, and ninety-two anti-cigarette bills are pending in twenty-eight states. Young women are expelled from college for smoking cigarettes.[70]

1921   · The Council of the American Medical Association refuses to confirm the Association's 1917 Resolution on alcohol. In the first six months after the enactment of the Volstead Act, more than 15,000 physicians and 57,000 druggists and drug manufacturers apply for licenses to prescribe and sell liquor.[71]

1921   Alfred C. Prentice, M.D., a member of the Committee on Narcotic Drugs of the American Medical Association, declares: "Public opinion regarding the vice of drug addiction has been deliberately and consistently corrupted through propaganda in both the medical and lay press. . . . The shallow pretense that drug addiction is a 'disease' . . . has been asserted and urged in volumes of 'literature' by self-styled 'specialists.' "[72]

1924   The manufacture of heroin is prohibited in the United States.

1925   Robert A. Schless: "I believe that most drug addiction today is due directly to the Harrison Anti-Narcotic Act, which forbids the sale of narcotics without a physician's prescription. . . . Addicts who are broke act as *agents provocateurs* for the peddlers, being rewarded by gifts of heroin or credit for supplies. The Harrison Act made the drug peddler, and the drug peddler makes drug addicts."[73]

1928   In a nationwide radio broadcast entitled "The Struggle of Mankind Against Its Deadliest Foe," celebrating the second annual Narcotic Education

Week, Richmond P. Hobson, prohibition crusader and anti-narcotics propagandist, declares: "Suppose it were announced that there were more than a million lepers among our people. Think what a shock the announcement would produce! Yet drug addiction is far more incurable than leprosy, far more tragic to its victims, and is spreading like a moral and physical scourge. . . . Most of the daylight robberies, daring hold-ups, cruel murders and similar crimes of violence are now known to be committed chiefly by drug addicts, who constitute the primary cause of our alarming crime wave. Drug addiction is more communicable and less curable than leprosy. . . . Upon the issue hangs the perpetuation of civilization, the destiny of the world, and the future of the human race."[74]

1928   It is estimated that in Germany one out of every hundred physicians is a morphine addict, consuming 0.1 gram of the alkaloid or more per day.[75]

1929   About one gallon of denatured industrial alcohol in ten is diverted into bootleg liquor. About forty Americans per million die each year from drinking illegal alcohol, mainly as a result of methyl (wood) alcohol poisoning.[76]

1930   The Federal Bureau of Narcotics is formed. Many of its agents, including its first commissioner, Harry J. Anslinger, are former prohibition agents.

1935   The American Medical Association passes a resolution declaring that "alcoholics are valid patients."[77]

1936   The Pan-American Coffee Bureau is organized at the first Pan-American Coffee Conference, in Bogotá, Colombia. A principal objective of the Bureau is "to formulate a co-operative effort for the promotion of increase in per capita consumption of coffee in the United States through the creation of a fund to conduct an educational and advertising campaign." During the first four-year period from the start of the Bureau's advertising (1938 to 1941), U.S. coffee consumption increases approximately 20 percent, while it takes twenty-four years (1914 to 1937) for another similar increase to occur.[78]

1937   Shortly before the passage of the Marijuana Tax Act, Commissioner Harry J. Anslinger writes: "How many murders, suicides, robberies, criminal assaults, hold-ups, burglaries, and deeds of maniacal insanity it [marijuana] causes each year, especially among the young, can only be conjectured."[79]

1937   The Marijuana Tax Act is enacted.

1938   Since the enactment of the Harrison Act in 1914, 25,000 physicians have been arraigned on narcotics charges, and 3,000 served penitentiary sentences.[80]

1938   Dr. Albert Hofmann, a chemist at Sandoz Laboratories in Basle, Switzerland, synthesizes LSD. Five years later he inadvertently ingests a small amount of it, and observes and reports its effects on himself.

1941   Generalissimo Chiang Kai-shek orders the complete suppression of the poppy: laws are enacted providing the death penalty for anyone guilty of cultivating the poppy, manufacturing opium, or offering it for sale.[81]

1943   Colonel J. M. Phalen, editor of the *Military Surgeon,* declares in an editorial entitled "The Marijuana Bugaboo": "The smoking of the leaves, flowers, and seeds of Cannabis sativa is no more harmful than the smoking of tobacco. . . . It is hoped that no witch hunt will be instituted in the military service over a problem that does not exist."[82]

1946	According to some estimates, there are 40,000,-000 opium smokers in China.[83]
1949	Ludwig von Mises, leading modern free-market economist and social philosopher: "Opium and morphine are certainly dangerous, habit-forming drugs. But once the principle is admitted that it is the duty of government to protect the individual against his own foolishness, no serious objections can be advanced against further encroachments. A good case could be made out in favor of the prohibition of alcohol and nicotine. And why limit the government's benevolent providence to the protection of the individual's body only? Is not the harm a man can inflict on his mind and soul even more disastrous than any bodily evils? Why not prevent him from reading bad books and seeing bad plays, from looking at bad paintings and statues and from hearing bad music? The mischief done by bad ideologies, surely, is much more pernicious, both for the individual and for the whole society, than that done by narcotic drugs."[84]
1951	According to United Nations estimates, there are approximately 200 million marijuana users in the world, the major places of use being India, Egypt, North Africa, Mexico, and the United States.[85]
1951	Twenty thousand pounds of opium, three hundred pounds of heroin, and various opium-smoking devices are publicly burned in Canton, China. Thirty-seven opium addicts are executed in the southwest of China.[86]
1954	Four-fifths of the French people questioned about wine assert that wine is "good for one's health," and one quarter hold that it is "indispensable." It is estimated that a third of the electorate in France receives all or part of its income from the production or sale of alcoholic beverages; and

that there is one outlet for the sale of alcohol for every forty-five inhabitants.[87]

1955   The Präsidium des Deutschen Ärztetages declares: "Treatment of the drug addict should be effected in the closed sector of a psychiatric institution. Ambulatory treatment is useless and in conflict, moreover, with principles of medical ethics." This view is quoted approvingly, as representative of the opinion of "most of the authors recommending commitment to an institution," by the World Health Organization in 1962.[88]

1955   The Shah of Iran prohibits the cultivation and use of opium, used in the country for thousands of years; the prohibition creates a flourishing illicit market in opium. In 1969 the prohibition is lifted, opium growing is resumed under state inspection, and more than 110,000 persons receive opium from physicians and pharmacies as "registered addicts."[89]

1956   The Narcotic Drug Control Act is enacted; it provides the death penalty, if recommended by the jury, for the sale of heroin to a person under eighteen by one over eighteen.[90]

1958   Ten percent of the arable land in Italy is under viticulture; two million people earn their living wholly or partly from the production or sale of wine.[91]

1960   The United States report to the United Nations Commission on Narcotic Drugs for 1960 states: "There were 44,906 addicts in the United States on 31 December 1960 . . ."[92]

1961   The United Nations' "Single Convention on Narcotic Drugs of 10 March 1961" is ratified. Among the obligations of the signatory states are the following: "Art. 42. Known users of drugs and persons charged with an offense under this Law may be committed by an examining magistrate to a nursing home. . . . Rules shall be also laid down for the treatment in such nursing homes of unconvicted drug addicts and dangerous alcoholics."[93]

1962   Supreme Court Justice William O. Douglas declares: "The addict is under compulsion not capable of management without outside help. . . . If addicts can be punished for their addiction, then the insane can also be punished for their insanity. Each has a disease and each must be treated as a sick person."[94]

1963   Mrs. Jean Nidetch, a formerly overweight housewife, incorporates Weight Watchers, an organization of diet clubs. By 1968, approximately 750,-000 persons join Weight Watchers.[95]

1963   Tobacco sales total $8.08 billion, of which $3.3 billion go to federal, state, and local governments in excise taxes. A news release from the tobacco industry proudly states: "Tobacco products pass across sales counters more frequently than anything else—except money."[96]

1964   The British Medical Association, in a Memorandum of Evidence to the Standing Medical Advisory Committee's Special Sub-committee on Alcoholism, declares: "We feel that in some very bad cases, compulsory detention in hospital offers the only hope of successful treatment. . . . We believe that some alcoholics would welcome compulsory removal and detention in hospital until treatment is completed."[97]

1964   An editorial in *The New York Times* calls attention to the fact that "the Government continues to be the tobacco industry's biggest booster. The Department of Agriculture lost $16 million in supporting the price of tobacco in the last fiscal year, and stands to lose even more because it has just raised the subsidy that tobacco growers will get on their 1964 crop. At the same time, the Food for Peace program is getting rid of surplus stocks of tobacco abroad."[98]

1966   Sen. Warren G. Magnuson makes public a program, sponsored by the Agriculture Department, to subsidize "attempts to increase cigarette consumption abroad. . . . The Department is paying Warner Brothers $106,000 to insert scenes designed to stimulate cigarette smoking in a travelogue for distribution in eight countries, and is also spending $210,000 to subsidize cigarette commercials in Japan, Thailand, and Austria." An Agriculture Department spokesman corroborates that "the two programs were prepared under a congressional authorization to expand overseas markets for U.S. farm commodities."[99]

1966   Congress enacts the Narcotic Addict Rehabilitation Act, inaugurating a federal civil commitment program for addicts.

1966   C. W. Sandman, Jr., chairman of the New Jersey Narcotic Drug Study Commission, declares that LSD is "the greatest threat facing the country today . . . more dangerous than the Vietnam War."[100]

1967   New York State's "Narcotics Addiction Control Program" goes into effect. It is estimated to cost $400 million in three years, and is hailed by Governor Rockefeller as "the start of an unending war . . ." Under the new law, judges are empowered to commit addicts for compulsory treatment for up to five years.[101]

1967   The tobacco industry in the United States spends an estimated $250 million on advertising smoking.[102]

1968   The U.S. tobacco industry has gross sales of $8 billion. Americans smoke 544 billion cigarettes.[103]

1968   Canadians buy almost 3 billion aspirin tablets and
               approximately 56 million standard doses of am-
               phetamines. About 556 million standard doses of
               barbiturates are also produced or imported for
               consumption in Canada.[104]

1968   Six to seven percent of all prescriptions written
               under the British National Health Service are for
               barbiturates; it is estimated that about 500,000
               Britons are regular users.[105]

1968   Abram Hoffer, M.D., and Humphry Osmond,
               M.D., claim that "strong evidence supporting the
               use of LSD in a treatment program for alcoholism
               comes from all parts of the world. It is one of the
               brightest hopes for the victims of a long neglected,
               little understood disease."[106]

1968   Addiction to heroin is treated in Britain with the
               implantation of radioactive yttrium-90 in the
               brain.[107]

1968   Brooklyn councilman Julius S. Moskowitz charges
               that the work of New York City's Addiction Serv-
               ices Agency, under its retiring Commissioner, Dr.
               Efren Ramirez, was a "fraud," and that "not a
               single addict has been cured."[108]

1969   The legal alcoholic beverage industry in the U.S.
               has a gross sale of $12 billion—more than is spent
               on education, medical care, and religion com-
               bined. Americans consume approximately 650
               million gallons of distilled spirits, 100 million bar-
               rels and 6 billion cans of beer, 200 million gallons
               of wine, 100 million gallons of moonshine (il-
               legal whiskey), and an unknown amount of home-
               made wine and beer.[109]

1969   The world production of tobacco is 4.6 million
               metric tons, with the U.S., U.S.S.R., China, and
               Brazil as the leading producers; of wine, 275 mil-
               lion hectoliters, with Italy, France, and Spain as
               the leading producers; of beer, 595 million hecto-

liters, with the U.S., Germany, and the U.S.S.R. as the leading producers; of cigarettes, 2,500 billion, with the U.S., U.S.S.R., and Japan as the leading producers.[110]

1969 U.S. production and value of some medicinal chemicals: barbiturates: 800,000 pounds, $2.5 million; aspirin (exclusive of salicylic acid): 37 million pounds, value "withheld to avoid disclosing figures for individual producers"; salicylic acid: 13 million pounds, $13 million; tranquilizers: 1.5 million pounds, $7 million.[111]

1969 A report issued by the United Nations Food and Agriculture Organization discloses that, despite warnings about the deleterious effects of smoking on health, the consumption of cigarettes throughout the world is growing at the annual rate of 70 billion cigarettes. The United States exports tobacco leaf to 113 countries; tobacco accounts for one-third of all Greek exports, and one-fifth of the Turkish exports.[112]

1969 The parents of 6,000 secondary-school pupils in Clifton, New Jersey, are sent letters by the Board of Education asking permission to conduct saliva tests on their children to determine whether or not they use marijuana.[113]

1970 New York State assemblyman Alfred D. Lerner introduces a bill to ban the sale of candy cigarettes in New York State, "to de-glamorize smoking in the eyes of children."[114]

1970 Dr. Alan F. Guttmacher, president of Planned Parenthood–World Population, declares that the Pill is "a prophylaxis against one of the gravest sociomedical illnesses—unwanted pregnancy."[115]

1970 Dr. Albert Szent-Györgyi, Nobel Laureate in Medicine and Physiology, in reply to being asked what he would do if he were twenty today: "I would share with my classmates rejection of the whole world as it is—all of it. Is there any point in studying and work? Fornication—at least that is something good. What else is there to do? Fornicate and take drugs against this terrible strain of idiots who govern the world."[116]

1970   Per capita cigarette smoking increases, "from 3,993 for each smoker in 1969, to 5,030 for each one in 1970."[117]

1970   Tobacco consumption is increasing rapidly in Russia: "In 1960, Soviet retail stores sold $1.5 billion rubles of tobacco products. By 1968, the figure had risen to $2.4 billion, more than a 50 per cent rise."[118]

1970   Calculated on the basis of the taxes paid on alcoholic beverages, the lowest consumption per year per person in the drinking-age population is in Arkansas, with 1.35 gallons of distilled spirits, 0.86 gallons of wine, and 16.20 gallons of beer, for a total consumption of absolute alcohol per capita per year of 1.47 gallons; and the highest consumption is in the District of Columbia, with 10.39 gallons of distilled spirits, 5.24 gallons of wine, and 31.48 gallons of beer, for a total of absolute alcohol per person of 6.94 gallons. This rate is higher than that in any other country, the next-highest rate being in France, with a per capita absolute alcohol consumption of 6.53 gallons; the comparable rates are 4.01 gallons for Italy, 3.39 gallons for Switzerland, 2.61 gallons for the United States, and 0.82 gallons for Israel.[119]

1970   Having passed both Houses of Congress by unanimous votes, the "Comprehensive Alcohol Abuse and Alcoholism Prevention, Treatment, and Rehabilitation Act of 1970" is signed into law by President Nixon.

1970   According to a release of the U. S. Department

of Health, Education, and Welfare, "An estimated
1.3 billion prescriptions were filled in 1970, at a
consumer cost of $5.6 billion. Of these, 17 per
cent, or 214 million, were for psychotherapeutic
drugs (anti-anxiety agents, anti-depressants, anti-
psychotics, stimulants, hypnotics, and seda-
tives)."[120]

1970   Henri Nargeolet, chief of the Central Service of
Pharmacy and Drugs of the French Ministry of
Public Health and Social Security, declares, after
the French National Assembly adopts a new anti-
drug bill, that "drug addiction will henceforth be
considered as a contagious disease in France, as
are alcoholism and venereal disease."[121]

1970   The world production of tobacco is 4.7 million
metric tons; of wine, 300 million hectoliters; of
beer, 630 million hectoliters; of cigarettes, 2,600
billion.[122]

1971   President Nixon declares that "America's Public Enemy No. 1 is drug abuse." In a message to
Congress, the President calls for the creation of
a Special Action Office of Drug Abuse Prevention.[123]

1971   New York City Mayor John Lindsay testifies before a House subcommittee that "with intensive
research it should be feasible to develop an inoc-
ulation against heroin which would be administered to youngsters in the same way as vaccines
against smallpox, polio, measles . . . and only a
Federal scientific task force approaching the scale
proposed for cancer research can bring the sort
of breakthrough we need."[124]

1971   A survey of smoking habits and economics by the
Sunday Telegraph (London) reveals that: in
Spain, tobacco is a state monopoly, with annual
gross income last year at $210 million; in Italy, it
is also a state monopoly, with profits at $1.3 bil-

lion, or 8 percent of the total tax revenue; in Switzerland, government revenue from tobacco taxes was $60 million, or 5 percent of the total; in Norway, it was $70 million, or 3 percent of the total; and in Sweden, it was $350 million, or 2 percent of the total tax revenue.[125]

1971   On June 30, 1971, President Cevdet Sunay of Turkey decrees that all poppy cultivation and opium production will be forbidden beginning in the fall of 1972.[126]

1971   John N. Mitchell, Attorney General of the United States, declares: "I refer to the fact, acknowledged now by all professionals in the field, that alcoholism as such is not a legal problem—it is a health problem. More especially, simple drunkenness per se should not be handled as an offense subject to the processes of justice. It should be handled as an illness, subject to medical treatment. . . . [W]e know that it does little good to remove alcoholism from the purview of the law if you do not substitute a full-dress medical treatment—not only a detoxification process, but a thoroughgoing program aimed at recovery from the illness of alcoholism. Again, the program must include the closest cooperation and communication, starting at the top level, between the public health officials and law enforcement officials. The police must have an understanding that their role continues—not in an arresting capacity, but in one of helping subjects to the designated health centers, voluntarily if possible, involuntarily if necessary."[127]

1972   Myles J. Ambrose, Special Assistant Attorney General of the United States: "As of 1960, the Bureau of Narcotics estimated that we had somewhere in the neighborhood of 55,000 heroin addicts . . . they estimate now the figure to be 560,000 addicts."[128]

1972   The Bureau of Narcotic and Dangerous Drugs proposes restricting the use of barbiturates on the ground that they "are more dangerous than heroin."[129]

1972   The House votes 366 to 0 to authorize "a $1 billion, three-year federal attack on drug abuse."[130]

1972   At the Bronx House of Correction, out of a total of 780 inmates, approximately 400 are given tranquilizers such as Valium, Elavil, Thorazine, and Librium. " 'I think they [the inmates] would be doing better without some of the medication,' said Capt. Robert Brown, a correction officer. He said that in a way the medications made his job harder . . . rather than becoming calm, he said, an inmate who had become addicted to his medication 'will do anything when he can't get it.' "[131]

1972   On December 23, Reuters reports: "The Italian Government has approved a law under which drug addicts would be treated as sick people rather than criminals. A government statement said that under the new law . . . an addict would face minimal penalties and none at all if he agreed to submit to medical treatment."[132]

1972   In England, the pharmacy cost of heroin is $.04 per grain (60 mg.), or $.00067 per mg. In the United States, the street price is $30 to $90 per grain, or $.50 to $1.50 per mg.[133]

1972   President Nixon calls "drug abuse the nation's public enemy No. 1," and proposes federal spending of $600 million for fiscal 1973 "to battle the drug problem from poppy-grower to pusher."[134]

1973   According to *Barron's,* the weekly financial newspaper, health care is the largest industry in the United States. In fiscal 1973, Americans will spend $90 billion on health care, compared with $76.4 billion for defense. Only 32 percent of the total bill is paid for directly, 30 percent coming from insurance companies, and 38 percent from the government.[135]

1973   A nationwide Gallup poll reveals that 67 percent of the adults interviewed "support the proposal of New York Governor Nelson Rockefeller that all sellers of hard drugs be given life imprisonment without the possibility of parole." Among the typical comments cited by Gallup: "The seller of drugs is not human . . . therefore he should be removed from society."[136]

1973   Myles J. Ambrose, Special Attorney General in charge of the Office for Drug Abuse, defending the methods used by his agents in apprehending alleged drug abusers: "Drug people are the very vermin of humanity. . . . Occasionally we must adopt their dress and tactics."[137]

1973   "Citing opposition from 'misguided softliners,'" Governor Rockefeller signs into law "the toughest anti-drug program in the nation." He also requests the legislature "'to provide funds to nearly double the state's narcotics treatment facilities.' . . . The new law calls for mandatory minimum jail terms for drug pushers and possessors but will allow parole under lifetime supervision."[138]

1973   Michael R. Sonnenreich, Executive Director of the National Commission on Marijuana and Drug Abuse, declares: "About four years ago we spent a total of $66.4 million for the entire federal effort in the drug abuse area. . . . This year we have spent $796.3 million, and the budget estimates that have been submitted indicate that we will exceed the $1 billion mark. When we do so, we become, for want of a better term, a drug abuse industrial complex."[139]

Addendum to the Appendix

The "War on Drugs"
1974-1984

Traditionally, in Judeo-Christian cultures, sexual behavior has constituted the core concern of morality. This reigning role of sex in the moral calculus of our forebears is exemplified by the parable of the Fall. Although that act has always been interpreted (no doubt correctly) as referring to sexual intercourse between man and woman, it is important to remember that the Bible writers did not name that "crime" directly but only alluded to it through the metaphor of partaking of the Forbidden Fruit. Inasmuch as that primal act of defiance of God's authority clearly transcends the image through which it was for so long mediated, it is perhaps not surprpsing that drugs have now replaced sex in the grand morality play of human existence. No longer are men, women and children tempted, corrupted, and ruined by the irresistibly sweet pleasures of sex; instead, they are tempted, corrupted, and ruined by the irresistibly sweet pleasures of drugs. Thus, youth's defiance of adult authority and, more generally, man's defiance of society's demands for conformity, is now enacted through ceremonies of drug use, called "drug abuse"; and the celebration of the legitimacy and power of medical, parental, and societal authority is now enacted through the counter-ceremonies of drug controls, called the "war on drugs."

I have put together this Addendum partly to bring the synoptic history presented in the Appendix up to date, and partly to re-emphasize, once again, the essentially ritual character of the "war on drugs."

1974   An article in the *American Journal of Psychiatry* advocates treating alcoholism in American Indians with peyote (an illicit drug), because it "offers the alcoholic Indian both occupational and cultural therapy including participation in the services of the Native American Church (peyote meetings)."[140]

1975   Jerome H. Jaffe, former top White House drug abuse official, "urge[s] that people who smoke a pack [of cigarettes] a day or more be described as suffering from a 'compulsive smoking disorder,' " and explains to a Third World Conference on Smoking and Health, that "a new term—'compulsive smoking syndrome'—has been proposed as a disorder to be listed in the Diagnostic and Statistical Manual of the American Psychiatric Association."[141]

1976   Rosalynn Carter, wife of Democratic Presidential nominee Jimmy Carter, tells the press that "her three grown sons 'have smoked marijuana—they told me they did.' . . . Mrs. Carter's statements, reminiscent of some made by Betty Ford, were consistent with her previous position that marijuana should be decriminalized but not legalized, a Carter aide said."[142]

1977   A British story on the war against laetrile reports that: "U.S. Federal Marshals last month seized 50 tons of apricot stones . . . probably the largest seizure of an illegal drug base in the history of U.S. law enforcement."[143]

1977   The Labor Department directs employers with federal contracts "to take 'affirmative action' to hire alcoholics and drug abusers . . . [A]lcoholics and drug abusers are covered by the 1973 Rehabilitation Act, which protects 'handicapped people' against job discrimination. 'Employers who fail to consider qualified alcoholics and drug abusers for employment because of their handicap are clearly violating the law,' Mr. Elisburg [Donald Elisburg, assistant secretary of labor for employment standards] said."[144]

1978   Peter Bourne, special assistant to President Carter and director of the White House Office of Drug Abuse Policy, writes an illegal prescription for Quaaludes for one of his aides and is forced to resign. On leaving the White House, he tells the press that there is a "high incidence of marijuana use . . . [and] occasional use of cocaine" by members of the White House staff.[145]

1979   In Jacksonville, Florida, actress Linda Blair is "ordered to become a crusader against drug abuse as part of her probation after pleading guilty to a federal misdemeanor charge of conspiracy to possess cocaine."[146]

1980   Dr. Lee Macht, a Harvard professor of psychiatry, who treated David Kennedy, admits that "he prescribed drugs illegally to the 24-year-old nephew of Senator Edward Kennedy. . . . [He is] fined $1,000 and . . . his license to prescribe Class 2 drugs [is] suspended for at least one year. The Middlesex County assistant district attorney said that at least 50 prescriptions over a 2½ -year period were written for the young Kennedy, involving the drugs Percodan, Diluadid . . . and Quaaludes."[147]

1980   At a conference in New York City announcing the creation of a "new commission to fight the drug menace," Governor Hugh Carey declares: "The epidemic of gold-chain snatching in the city is the result of a Russian design to wreck America by flooding the nation with deadly heroin. . . . [If the Russians] were using nerve gas on us, we'd certainly call out the troops. This is more insidious than nerve gas. Nerve gas passes off. This doesn't. It kills. I am not overstating the case."[148]

1980   Japan agrees to provide concessions to the U.S. tobacco industry "that could increase sales there from $35 million to about $350 million [annually]." In a new trade agreement announced by Steve Lande, assistant U.S. trade representative for bilateral affairs, Japan would "reduce tariffs on cigarettes . . . increase the number of retailers selling imported tobacco products . . . [and] permit U.S. companies to advertise in Japan."[149]

1980   Christopher Lawford, son of Peter Lawford and Patricia Kennedy Lawford and nephew of Senator Edward Kennedy, is arraigned in Boston on a charge of possessing heroin.[150]

1981   Responding to questions concerning the problems created by the PCB contamination of a state office building in Binghamton, New York, Governor Hugh Carey volunteers "to drink a glass of PCBs . . . to demonstrate that the building was safe. 'I offer here and now [said Carey] to walk into Binghamton or any part of that building and swallow an entire glass of PCBs. . . . If I had a couple of willing hands and a few vacuum cleaners, I'd clean that building myself.' "[151]

1981   Janet Cooke, a Washington Post reporter, wins a Pulitzer Prize for her story titled "8-Year-Old Heroin Addict Lives for a Fix," which turns out to be a complete fabrication. The *Post's* Executive Editor, Benjamin Bradlee, attributes the fraud to mental illness, explaining to an interviewer: "We're going to take care of her. We're going to see that she has professional help."[152]

1981   *Time* magazine reports on Project Pearl, an effort to smuggle 1 million contraband Chinese-language Bibles into mainland China. The project is backed by a Dutch-based evangelical missionary organization called "Brother Andrew International," specializing "in smuggling Bibles into Communist countries." The 1 million Chinese Bibles are produced by Thomas Nelson Publishers at a cost of 1.4 million, weigh 232 tons, and are shipped to Hong Kong in 1980 for distribution to smugglers. Publicity about the project has "inspired calls from potential donors willing to finance massive new Bible-smuggling ventures to China or behind the Iron Curtain."[153]

1981   In an effort to curb the revival if Islamic fundamentalism, the Turkish government bans "the wearing of head kerchiefs by female students and teachers in schools."[154]

1982   The U.S. Supreme Court upholds the constitutionality of "a 40-year prison sentence imposed on a Virginia man for possession and distribution of nine ounces of marijuana, worth about $200. The unsigned decision . . . reversed rulings by two lower Federal courts that the sentence was so harsh in proportion to the crime as to violate the Eighth Amendment's prohibition against cruel and unusual punishment."[155]

1982   In Tucson, Arizona, a 21-year-old man is sentenced to two years in prison for sniffing paint, under an Arizona law that reads: "A person shall not knowingly breathe, inhale, or drink a vapor-releasing substance containing a toxic substance." Police and prosecutors are said to favor the law because "intoxicated sniffers can grow violent."[156]

1982   An editorial in the New York Post declares: "Drugs are now the scourge of our society. . . . [Parents] should ask their children this question: 'What did John Belushi have in common with Elvis Presley, Freddie Prinze, Janis Joplin, Jimi Hendrix, Billie Holiday, Lenny Bruce, Frankie Lymon, Miguel Berrios, and Charlie Parker? Answer: They all took

218   APPENDIX

drugs and they all killed themselves doing so.' "¹⁵⁷

1983   In an interview in *The Washington Times*, Senator Barry Goldwater volunteers the information that his son, former Representative Barry Goldwater, Jr., "smoked marijuana; he admitted that. He sniffed a little coke (cocaine); he admitted that."¹⁵⁸

1983   The Drug Enforcement Agency acknowledges using entrapment in fighting the war on drugs. "Federal drug agents seeking to draw out potential producers of hallucinogens and other illicit drugs have been operating bogus chemical companies that sell materials and instructions for the manufacture of such dangerous drugs. Then they arrest their customers. . . . The tactic . . . has already lead to convictions . . ."¹⁵⁹

1983   John V. Lindsay, Jr., son of former New York City Mayor John V. Lindsay, is sentenced to six months in prison for selling three grains of cocaine to an undercover agent.¹⁶⁰

1983   Dr. Andrew Rynne, a physician in County Kildare, Ireland, pleads guilty "to supplying condoms to a patient illegally [on a weekend]" and is fined ℔ 500.¹⁶¹

1983   Shrimp farmers in Israel succeed in "growing" the crustacean in commercial quantities. "Shrimp sales mean hard currency and they are one of Israel's up and coming export industries. . . . The Kibbutzniks in northern Israel have promised the rabbis that their shrimp will only be sold abroad."¹⁶²

1984   In Rapid City, South Dakota, Robert F. Kennedy, Jr., a former Assistant District Attorney in New York City, pleads guilty to a felony charge of possessing heroin.¹⁶³

1984   Commenting on David Kennedy's suicide (with an overdose of cocaine, Demerol and Mellaril), New York City Mayor Edward Koch declares: " '[Kennedy] was killed by a drug pusher. I believe the person who sold him those drugs is guilty of murder.' . . . Koch said he wanted to see capital punishment for such crimes on a national level."[164]

1984   School officials order the suspension of any Wilmington, Massachusetts, High School student "caught with drugs, including aspirin and over-the-counter medications." The rule, "written with the help of the U.S. Drug Enforcement Administration . . . requires students to store drugs and pills in the school clinic. Robert Stutmant, head of the Boston office of the DEA, explained that the ruling was required because 'a drop of LSD can be concealed in an aspirin tablet . . .' "[165]

References

Epigram, page vii

Edmund Burke, A Letter from Mr. Burke to a Member of the National Assembly in Answer to Some Objections to His Book on French Affairs, 1791, in *The Works of the Right Honorable Edmund Burke*, Vol. 3, p. 315.

INTRODUCTION

1. See also Thomas Szasz, *Ideology and Insanity* and *The Age of Madness.*
2. See Gilbert Ryle, *The Concept of Mind.*

CHAPTER 1
The Discovery of Drug Addiction

1. See Thomas Szasz, The ethics of addiction, *Harper's Magazine*, April 1972, pp. 74–79, and Bad habits are not diseases, *Lancet*, 2:83–84 (July 8), 1972.
2. See, especially, Thomas Szasz, *The Myth of Mental Illness,* and *Ideology and Insanity.*
3. See Karl Menninger, *The Vital Balance,* pp. 419–489.
4. Ibid., p. 474.
5. Gregory Zilboorg, *A History of Medical Psychology,* pp. 591–606.
6. Jerome H. Jaffe, "Drug Addiction and Drug Abuse," in Louis Goodman and Alfred Gilman (Eds.), *The Pharmacological Basis of Therapeutics,* Fourth Edition, p. 276.
7. In this connection, see Thomas Szasz, *Law, Liberty, and Psychiatry* and *Psychiatric Justice.*
8. Philip H. Abelson, Death from heroin (editorial), *Science,* 168:1289 (June 12), 1970.
9. Jared Stout, New drug offers hope: May immunize heroin addicts, *Syracuse Herald-Journal,* Dec. 23, 1971, p. 1.
10. Boyce Rensenberger, Amphetamines used by a physician to lift moods of famous patients, *The New York Times,* Dec. 4, 1972, pp. 1 and 34.
11. John A. Hamilton, Hooked on histrionics, *The New York Times,* Feb. 12, 1973, p. 27.
12. Black leaders demand stiff drug penalties, *Human Events,* Feb. 17, 1973, p. 3.
13. Ibid.
14. William F. Buckley, Jr., Rockefeller's proposal, *Syracuse Post-Standard,* Feb. 15, 1973, p. 5.
15. Thomas Adams, Hanley urges stiffer penalties for drug abusers, *Syracuse Herald-Journal,* March 23, 1968, p. 2.
16. Steven Jonas, Dealing with drugs (letter to the editor), *The New York Times,* Jan. 12, 1973, p. 30.
17. See Thomas Szasz, *Ideology and Insanity,* especially pp. 218–245; and *The Age of Madness.*

CHAPTER 2
The Scapegoat as Drug and the Drug as Scapegoat

1. How the new drug laws affect you, *Syracuse Post-Standard*, Aug. 20, 1973, p. 5.
2. Ibid.
3. Ibid.
4. Jane Ellen Harrison, *Epilegomena to the Study of Greek Religion and Themis*, p. xvii.
5. Ibid.
6. Ibid.
7. Ibid.
8. James George Frazer, *The Golden Bough*, p. 579.
9. Ibid.
10. John Cuthbert Lawson, *Modern Greek Folklore and Ancient Greek Religion*, p. 355.
11. Gilbert Murray, *The Rise of the Greek Epic*, pp. 11–12.
12. Ibid., p. 12.
13. Martin P. Nilsson, *A History of Greek Religion*, p. 87.
14. Murray, op. cit., pp. 12–13.
15. Ibid., p. 14.
16. W. R. Paton, The pharmakoi and the story of the Fall, *Revue Archéologique*, 3:51–57, 1907.

CHAPTER 3
Medicine: The Faith of the Faithless

1. Kenneth Burke, Interaction: III. Dramatism, in David L. Sills (Ed.), *International Encyclopedia of the Social Sciences*, Vol. 7, p. 450.
2. Ibid., p. 451.
3. See Thomas Szasz, *Ideology and Insanity*.
4. See Edmund Wilson, The lexicon of prohibition (1927), in *The American Earthquake*, pp. 89–91.
5. Mary Douglas, *Purity and Danger*, p. 153.
6. See Marston Bates, *Gluttons and Libertines*.
7. Douglas, op. cit., p. 41.
8. Ibid., p. 42.
9. *Deuteronomy*, 14:3.
10. Douglas, op. cit., Chapter 3.
11. *Leviticus*, 21:16–21.
12. Douglas, op. cit., p. 68.

CHAPTER 4
Communions, Holy and Unholy

1. Matthew, 26:26–29.
2. Transubstantiation, *Encyclopaedia Britannica* (1949), Vol. 22, p. 417.
3. Genesis, 9:20.
4. Ibid., 14:18–19.

5. Exodus, 29:38, 40.
6. Leviticus, 23:13; Numbers, 15:5.
7. Matthew, 26:26–29.
8. John, 2:1–11.
9. Quoted in Edward M. Brecher et al., *Licit and Illicit Drugs*, p. 398.
10. Solomon H. Snyder, *Uses of Marijuana*, p. 20.
11. Quoted in ibid.
12. Ibid.
13. See Thomas Szasz, The role of the counterphobic mechanism in addiction, *Journal of the American Psychoanalytic Association*, 6:309–325, 1958.
14. See Chapter 12; also Thomas Szasz, The ethics of addiction, *Harper's Magazine*, April 1972, pp. 74–79.
15. Keith Thomas, *Religion and the Decline of Magic*, p. 17.
16. Ibid., p. 18.
17. Ibid., p. 19.
18. Ibid.
19. Ibid.
20. Ibid., p. 20.
21. Ibid.
22. Tennessee Williams, Interview, *Playboy*, April 1973, pp. 69–84; p. 76.
23. Ibid., p. 82.
24. Neil McCafrey, Letter to the editor, *National Review*, Feb. 2, 1973, p. 346.
25. Fox Butterfield, Laos' opium country resisting drug laws, *The New York Times*, Oct. 16, 1972, p. 12.
26. Ibid.
27. Ibid.
28. Ibid.
29. Henry Kamm, They shoot opium smugglers in Iran, but . . . , *The New York Times Magazine*, Feb. 11, 1973, pp. 42–45; p. 44.
30. Ibid.
31. Ibid.
32. Ibid.
33. Ibid., p. 45.
34. Ibid.
35. Ibid.
36. Ibid., p. 44.
37. See Thomas Szasz, *The Manufacture of Madness*, Chapter 11.
38. Art Linkletter, How do I tell if my child is hooked? *Syracuse Post-Standard*, March 3, 1970, p. 16.
39. Ira Mothner, How can you tell if your child is taking drugs? *Look*, Jan. 7, 1970, p. 42.
40. Henry Sutton, Drugs: Ten years to doomsday? *Saturday Review*, Nov. 14, 1970, pp. 18–21, 59–61.
41. Ibid., p. 19.
42. Ibid., p. 60.
43. Ibid.
44. Jerome H. Jaffe and Myles J. Ambrose, Administration's drive against drugs (letter to the editor), *The New York Times*, Oct. 7, 1972, p. 28.

45. Marion K. Sanders, Addicts and zealots, *Harper's Magazine*, June 1970, pp. 71–80; p. 71.
46. Bartenders in Milwaukee almost double in 2 years, *The New York Times*, Dec. 13, 1972, p. 22.

CHAPTER 5
Licit and Illicit Healing

1. In this connection, see, for example, Thomas R. Forbes, *The Midwife and the Witch*, especially pp. 129–130; Christina Hole, *Witchcraft in England*, pp. 129–130; Max Marwick (Ed.), *Witchcraft and Sorcery;* and John Middleton (Ed.), *Magic Witchcraft, and Curing.*
2. Jules Michelet, *Satanism and Witchcraft* (1862), p. 77.
3. Pennethorne Hughes, *Witchcraft*, p. 202.
4. Quoted in Michelet, op. cit., p. xi.
5. Quoted in Margaret A. Murray, *The Witch-Cult in Western Europe* (1921), p. 279.
6. Ibid., pp. 279–280.
7. Hughes, op. cit., p. 129.
8. Howard W. Haggard, *Devils, Drugs, and Doctors*, p. 73.
9. Michelet, op. cit., p. xix.
10. Excerpts from message by Governor Rockefeller on the State of the State, *The New York Times*, Jan. 4, 1973, p. 28.
11. See Charles Mackay, *Extraordinary Popular Delusions and the Madness of Crowds* (1841, 1852).
12. William E. Farrell, Governor's plan on drug abuse, *The New York Times*, Feb. 2, 1973, p. 13.
13. Ibid.
14. Ibid.
15. Ibid.
16. Ibid.
17. Editorial, Police as pushers, *The New York Times*, Dec. 26, 1972, p. 32.
18. Farrell, op. cit.
19. Ibid.
20. Ibid.
21. Editorial, Drug sidelines profitable, *Syracuse Herald-Journal*, Jan. 31, 1973, p. 14.
22. Francis X. Clines, Flexibility urged in narcotics case, *The New York Times*, Feb. 6, 1973, p. 29.

CHAPTER 6
Opium and Orientals

1. *The Chinese Exclusion Case*, 130 U.S. 581, 1889.
2. David I. Macht, The history of opium and some of its preparations and alkaloids, *Journal of the American Medical Association*, 64:477–481 (Feb. 6), 1915; p. 477.
3. John Ingersoll, quoted in U.S. urges "bold new" efforts by U.N. body on narcotics abuse, *The New York Times*, Jan. 13, 1970, p. 11.

4. See Chapter 10.
5. Herbert Hill, Anti-Oriental agitation and the rise of working-class racism, *Society*, 10:43–54 (Jan.–Feb.), 1973; p. 51.
6. Ibid., p. 52.
7. Ibid., p. 46.
8. Ibid.
9. Ibid., p. 52.
10. Edward M. Brecher et al., *Licit and Illicit Drugs*, p. 42.
11. Ibid., p. 43.
12. Ibid., p. 44.
13. See Helmut Schoeck, *Envy*.
14. Ernest Jones, *The Life and Work of Sigmund Freud*, Vol. 1, p. 80.
15. Ibid., p. 81.
16. Ibid., p. 82.
17. Ibid., p. 81.
18. See Chapter 7.
19. Quoted in Brecher et al., op. cit., p. 34.
20. Ibid.
21. Ibid.
22. Ibid., p. 35.
23. Quoted in Maurice B. Strauss (Ed.), *Familiar Medical Quotations*, p. 139.
24. See Chapter 10.
25. See, for example, Rufus King, *The Drug Hang-up*, p. 18.
26. Genesis, 2:15–17.
27. Ibid., 3:4–5.
28. Ibid., 3:14–19.

CHAPTER 7
Drugs and Devils

1. Malcolm X: *The Autobiography of Malcolm X*, front cover.
2. Jean-Paul Sartre, *Saint Genet*.
3. Malcolm X, op. cit., p. 387.
4. Ibid., p. 134.
5. Ibid., p. 138.
6. Ibid., p. 150.
7. Ibid., p. 153.
8. Ibid.
9. Ibid., p. 155.
10. Ibid., p. 156.
11. Ibid., p. 159.
12. Ibid., p. 163.
13. Ibid.
14. Ibid., p. 193.
15. Ibid., p. 221.
16. Ibid., p. 225.
17. Ibid., p. 226.
18. See, for example, Phyllis Chesler, *Women and Madness*.

19. Thomas Szasz, *The Manufacture of Madness*, Chapter 9.
20. Ibid., p. 153.
21. Ibid., p. 155.
22. Malcolm X, op. cit., p. xi.
23. Ibid., p. 164.
24. Ibid., p. 165.
25. Ibid., p. 166.
26. Ibid., p. 167.
27. Ibid., p. 259.
28. Ibid.
29. Ibid., p. 260.
30. Ibid., p. 261.
31. Alfred C. Prentice, The problem of the narcotic drug addict, *Journal of the American Medical Association*, 76:1551–1556 (June 4), 1921; p. 1553.
32. Malcolm X, op. cit., p. 384.
33. Ibid., p. 276.
34. Ibid., p. 262.

CHAPTER 8
Food Abuse and Foodaholism

1. H. R. Hays, *The Dangerous Sex*, especially Chapter 4.
2. Wilmer A. Asher, Bariatrics: Struggling for recognition, *Medical Opinion*, 1:20–21, 28–31 (Dec.), 1972, p. 28.
3. Ibid., pp. 20–21.
4. Harold A. Harper, Foreword, in Nancy L. Wilson (Ed.), *Obesity*, p. vii.
5. Joseph M. Fee et al., Obesity: A Gross National Product, in Wilson (Ed.), op. cit., pp. 239–245.
6. *Physicians' Desk Reference*, 27th Edition, p. 202.
7. Asher, op. cit., p. 21.
8. Natalie Allon, Group dieting rituals, *Society*, 10:36–42 (Jan.–Feb.), 1973; p. 37.
9. Ibid.
10. See Chapter 2.
11. Allon, op. cit., p. 37.
12. Ibid.
13. Charles Mackay, *Extraordinary Popular Delusions and the Madness of Crowds* (1841, 1852).
14. Fish and chips the enemy in USAF's 'Battle of the bulge,' *Syracuse Post-Standard*, Oct. 6, 1971, p. 11.
15. Off-limits, *Parade*, Jan. 6, 1972, p. 7.
16. See Thomas Szasz, *The Manufacture of Madness*, Chapter 11.
17. J. Howard Payne and Loren T. DeWind, Surgical treatment of obesity, *American Journal of Surgery*, 118:141–147 (Aug.), 1969; p. 146.
18. Jack M. Farris, in ibid., p. 147.
19. Ibid.
20. Harry H. LeVeen, Comments, in A. Bertrand Brill et al., Changes in body composition after jejunoileal bypass in morbidly obese patients, *American Journal of Surgery*, 123:49–56 (Jan.), 1972; p. 55.
21. Dead end, *Time*, Apr. 24, 1972, p. 65.

CHAPTER 9
Missionary Medicine

1. See especially Thomas Szasz, *Ideology and Insanity* and *The Manufacture of Madness.*
2. Thomas S. Blair, Habit indulgence in certain cactaceous plants among the Indians, *Journal of the American Medical Association,* 76:1033–1034 (April 9), 1921.
3. Edward M. Brecher et al., *Licit and Illicit Drugs,* p. 339.
4. Blair, op. cit., p. 1033.
5. Ibid., p. 1034.
6. Ibid.
7. Brecher, op. cit., p. 339.
8. Blair, op. cit., p. 1034.
9. Norman Taylor, The pleasant assassin, in David Solomon (Ed.), *The Marihuana Papers,* p. 41.
10. See Thomas Szasz, Scapegoating "military addicts," *Trans-action,* 9:4–6 (Jan.), 1972.
11. Manfred Guttmacher, *Sex Offenses,* p. 132.
12. Louis Goodman and Alfred Gilman, *The Pharmacological Basis of Therapeutics,* First Edition (1941), p. 186.
13. Ibid., Second Edition (1955), p. 216.
14. Ibid., Third Edition (1965), p. 247.
15. Ibid., Fourth Edition (1970), p. 237.
16. Editorial, Save school children now, *Syracuse Post-Standard,* Feb. 25, 1970, p. 4.
17. Governor Shafer calls LSD blinding hoax, *The New York Times,* Jan. 19, 1968, p. 22.
18. Ibid.
19. Senator denies LSD story hoax, *Syracuse Herald-Journal,* Jan. 19, 1968, p. 2.
20. Ibid.
21. Drug study chief: Raymond Philip Shafer, *The New York Times,* March 23, 1972, p. 18.
22. Henry L. Mencken, The cult of hope, in *Prejudices,* p. 86.

CHAPTER 10
Cures and Controls

1. See Chapter 2.
2. Thomas Szasz, *Law, Liberty, and Psychiatry,* p. 212.
3. In this connection, see David F. Musto, *The American Disease.*
4. Saccharin suspect in study, *The Evening Star and Daily News* (Washington), May 23, 1973, C-back page.
5. Ibid.
6. Quoted in David I. Macht, The history of opium and some of its preparations and alkaloids, *Journal of the American Medical Association,* 64:477–481 (Feb. 6), 1915; p. 479.
7. Quoted in Joseph Lyons, *Experience,* p. 136.
8. Quoted in William C. Hunter, *Bits of Old China* (1885), pp. 170–171.

9. See Thomas Szasz, *The Manufacture of Madness*, especially Chapters 9 and 11.
10. Atheistic Albania 'suffocates' all religious forms, *San Juan Star* (Puerto Rico), April 1, 1973, p. 10.
11. Ibid.
12. Czechs told religion bad for children, *Syracuse Post-Standard*, Feb. 21, 1972, p. 2.
13. This week, *National Review*, Aug. 31, 1973, p. 926.
14. See John Carlova, Are useful new drugs being bottled up by bureaucracy? *Medical Economics*, Aug. 6, 1973, pp. 94–106.
15. See Nancy Martin, Will they challenge your prescribing habits? *Medical Economics*, Aug. 20, 1973, pp. 31–38.
16. See David A. Green, The New York tax on prescriptions, *Physician's Management*, 13:15–17 (June), 1973.
17. *Commonwealth of Massachusetts v. Miller* (1972), quoted in *The Citation* (A.M.A.), 25:156–157 (Sept. 1), 1972.
18. Ibid., p. 157.
19. *U.S. v. Bartee* (1973), quoted in *The Citation* (A.M.A.), 27:135–136 (Aug. 15), 1973.
20. Ibid.
21. See Erich Goode, *Drugs in American Society*, p. 191.
22. Drug legislation, *Massachusetts Physician*, 31:33 (May), 1972.
23. Matthew, 26:52.

CHAPTER 11
Temptation and Temperance

1. See Jane Ellen Harrison, *Epilegomena to the Study of Greek Religion and Themis*, especially pp. 118–157.
2. Quoted in Burton Stevenson (Ed.), *The Macmillan Book of Proverbs, Maxims, and Famous Phrases*, p. 2291.
3. Ibid.
4. Ibid.
5. James, 1:12.
6. Stevenson, op. cit., p. 2292.
7. See Thomas Szasz, *The Second Sin*, pp. 63–66.
8. René Gillouin, *Man's Hangman Is Man*, p. 67.
9. See Thomas Szasz, *The Manufacture of Madness*, pp. 180–206.
10. Advertisement, *The New York Times Magazine*, Jan. 14, 1973, p. 57.
11. William O. Douglas, Concurring opinion, in *Robinson v. California*, 370 U.S. 660, 1962; pp. 671, 673.
12. Ibid., p. 670.
13. Peter Laurie, *Drugs*, p. 32.
14. Helmut Schoeck, *Envy*.

CHAPTER 12
The Control of Conduct

1. See Thomas Szasz, *The Second Sin*.
2. See, especially, Ludwig von Mises, *Human Action*.

3. See, for example, S. Auerbach, "Behavior control" is scored, *Miami Herald*, Dec. 28, 1972, p. 15-A.

APPENDIX
A Synoptic History of the Promotion and Prohibition of Drugs

1. Alfred R. Lindesmith, *Addiction and Opiates*, p. 207.
2. Joel Fort, *The Pleasure Seekers*, p. 14.
3. Ashley Montagu, The long search for euphoria, *Reflections*, 1:62–69 (May–June), 1966; p. 66.
4. W. F. Crafts et al., *Intoxicating Drinks and Drugs*, p. 5.
5. Quoted in Berton Roueché, *The Neutral Spirit*, pp. 150–151.
6. Quoted in Burton Stevenson (Ed.), *The Macmillan Book of Proverbs, Maxims, and Famous Phrases*, p. 2520.
7. Alfred R. Lindesmith, *The Addict and the Law*, p. 194.
8. Richard S. Storrs, *John Wycliffe and the English Bible* (1880), p. 21.
9. Quoted in Roueché, op. cit., p. 144.
10. Joseph H. Dahmus, *The Prosecution of John Wyclyf*, p. 119.
11. Ibid., p. 384.
12. Friedrich Heer, *The Intellectual History of Europe*, Vol. 2, p. 30.
13. William Shakespeare, *Second Part of King Henry the Fourth*, Act IV, Scene III, lines 133–136.
14. Griffith Edwards, Psychoactive substances, *The Listener*, March 23, 1972, pp. 360–363; p. 361.
15. Ibid.
16. Heer, op. cit., Vol. 2, p. 31.
17. Edward M. Brecher et al., *Licit and Illicit Drugs*, p. 212.
18. Quoted in Louis Goodman and Alfred Gilman, *The Pharmacological Basis of Therapeutics*, First Edition (1941), p. 186.
19. Roueché, op. cit., p. 27.
20. Edwards, op. cit., p. 361.
21. G. E. G. Catlin, *Liquor Control*, p. 14.
22. Ibid., p. 15.
23. Ibid., p. 14.
24. Eleanor Flexner, *Century of Struggle*, p. 13.
25. Quoted in S. S. Rosenberg (Ed.), *Alcohol and Health*, p. 26.
26. Crafts et al., op. cit., p. 9.
27. Quoted in ibid.
28. William A. Emboden, Jr., Ritual use of Cannabis Sativa L.: A historical-ethnographic survey, in Peter T. Furst (Ed.), *Flesh of the Gods*, pp. 214–236; pp. 227–228.
29. Catlin, op. cit., p. 113.
30. Quoted in Roueché, op. cit., p. 105.
31. Thomas De Quincey, *Confessions of an English Opium Eater* (1822), p. 143.
32. Montagu, op. cit., p. 67.
33. Quoted in Roueché, op. cit., pp. 87–88.
34. Emboden, op. cit., p. 228.

35. Abraham Lincoln, Temperance address, in Roy P. Basler (Ed.), *The Collected Works of Abraham Lincoln*, Vol. 1, p. 278.
36. Andrew Sinclair, *Era of Excess*, p. 92.
37. Quoted in David Musto, *The American Disease*, p. 258.
38. Sinclair, op. cit., p. 152.
39. Quoted in Musto, op. cit., pp. 71–72.
40. Quoted in Sinclair, op. cit., pp. 83–84.
41. Crafts et al., op. cit., p. 72.
42. Catlin, op. cit., p. 114.
43. Brecher et al., op. cit., p. 272.
44. Quoted in Ernest Jones, *The Life and Work of Sigmund Freud*, Vol. 1, p. 82.
45. Quoted in Musto, op. cit., p. 29.
46. Quoted in Norman Taylor, The pleasant assassin: The story of marihuana, in David Solomon (Ed.), *The Marihuana Papers*, pp. 31–47; p. 41.
47. Quoted in Roueché, op. cit., pp. 107–108.
48. Montagu, op. cit., p. 68.
49. Quoted in Crafts et al., op. cit., p. 14.
50. Quoted in Henry H. Lennard et al., Methadone treatment (letters), *Science*, 179:1078–1079 (March 16), 1973; p. 1079.
51. Sinclair, op. cit., p. 33.
52. Musto, op. cit., p. 15.
53. Quoted in ibid., p. 17.
54. Quoted in Lennard et al., op. cit., p. 1079.
55. Musto, op. cit., p. 3.
56. Quoted in Crafts et al., op. cit., p. 230.
57. Quoted in ibid.
58. Quoted in Lennard et al., op. cit., p. 1079.
59. Lawrence Kolb, *Drug Addiction*, pp. 145–146.
60. Musto, op. cit., p. 43.
61. Sinclair, op. cit., p. 180.
62. Ibid., p. 29.
63. Ibid., p. 61.
64. Ibid., pp. 117–118.
65. Quoted in ibid., p. 121.
66. David F. Musto, An historical perspective on legal and medical responses to substance use, *Villanova Law Review*, 18:808–817 (May), 1973; p. 816.
67. Fort, op. cit., p. 69.
68. Lindesmith, *The Addict and the Law*, p. 141.
69. Thomas S. Blair, Habit indulgence in certain cactaceous plants among the Indians, *Journal of the American Medical Association*, 76:1033–1034 (April 9), 1921; p. 1034.
70. Brecher et al., op. cit., p. 492.
71. Sinclair, op. cit., p. 410.
72. Alfred C. Prentice, The problem of the narcotic drug addict, *Journal of the American Medical Association*, 76:1551–1556 (June 4), 1921; p. 1553.
73. Robert A. Schless, The drug addict, *American Mercury*, 4:196–199 (Feb.), 1925; p. 198.

74. Quoted in Musto, *The American Disease*, p. 191.
75. Erich Hesse, *Narcotics and Drug Addiction*, p. 41.
76. Sinclair, op. cit., p. 201.
77. Quoted in Neil Kessel and Henry Walton, *Alcoholism*, p. 21.
78. Coffee, *Encyclopaedia Britannica* (1949), Vol. 5, p. 975A.
79. Quoted in John Kaplan, *Marijuana*, p. 92.
80. Kolb, op. cit., p. 146.
81. Lindesmith, *The Addict and the Law*, p. 198.
82. Quoted in ibid., p. 234.
83. Hesse, op. cit., p. 24.
84. Ludwig von Mises, *Human Action*, pp. 728–729.
85. Jock Young, *The Drugtakers*, p. 11.
86. Martin B. Margulies, China has no drug problem—why? *Parade*, Oct. 15, 1972, p. 22.
87. Kessel and Walton, op. cit., pp. 45, 73.
88. World Health Organization, *Treatment of Drug Addicts*, p. 5.
89. Henry Kamm, They shoot opium smugglers in Iran, but . . . , *The New York Times Magazine*, Feb. 11, 1973, pp. 42–45.
90. Lindesmith, *The Addict and the Law*, p. 26.
91. Kessel and Walton, op. cit., p. 46.
92. Lindesmith, *The Addict and the Law*, p. 100.
93. Charles Vaille, A model law for the application of the Single Convention on Narcotic Drugs, 1961, *United Nations Bulletin on Narcotics*, 21:1–12 (April–June), 1961.
94. William O. Douglas, Concurring opinion, *Robinson v. California*, 370 U.S., 671, 674, 1962.
95. Frederick J. Stare and Jelia C. Witschi, Diet books: Facts, fads, and frauds, *Medical Opinion*, 1:13–18 (Dec.), 1972.
96. Tobacco: After publicity surge, Surgeon General's Report seems to have little enduring effect, *Science*, 145:1021–1022 (Sept. 4), 1964; p. 1021.
97. Quoted in Kessel and Walton, op. cit., p. 126.
98. Editorial, Bigger agricultural subsidies . . . even for tobacco, *The New York Times*, Feb. 1, 1964, p. 22.
99. Edwin B. Haakinson, Senator shocked at U.S. try to hike cigarette use abroad, *Syracuse Herald-American*, Jan. 9, 1966, p. 2.
100. Quoted in Brecher et al., op. cit., p. 369.
101. Murray Schumach, Plan for addicts will open today: Governor hails start, *The New York Times*, April 1, 1967, p. 35.
102. Editorial, It depends on you, *Health News* (New York State), 45:1 (March), 1968.
103. Fort, op. cit., p. 21.
104. Canadian Government's Commission of Inquiry, *The Non-Medical Uses of Drugs*, p. 184.
105. Young, op. cit., p. 25.
106. Abram Hoffer and Humphry Osmond, *New Hope for Alcoholics*, p. 15.
107. Christine Doyle, Radio-active seeds in brain cure pop singer's addiction, *The Observer* (London), July 7, 1968, p. 1.
108. Charles G. Bennett, Addiction agency called a "fraud," *The New York Times*, Dec. 11, 1968, p. 47.

109. Fort, op. cit., pp. 14–15.
110. United Nations, *Statistical Yearbook, 1970*, pp. 154, 251, 252, 228.
111. *Statistical Abstracts of the United States, 1971*, 92nd Annual Edition, p. 75.
112. Use of cigarettes found on increase throughout the world, *The New York Times*, Oct. 1, 1969, p. 14.
113. Saliva tests asked for Jersey youths on marijuana use, *The New York Times*, Apr. 11, 1969, p. 32.
114. Candy cigs ban asked, *Syracuse Post-Standard*, Jan. 28, 1970, p. 1.
115. Alan F. Guttmacher, The pill trial, *Time*, March 9, 1970, p. 32.
116. Albert Szent-Györgyi, in *The New York Times*, Feb. 20, 1970, quoted in Mary Breastead, *Oh! Sex Education!*, p. 359.
117. The nation, *American Medical News*, Jan. 11, 1971, p. 2.
118. Bernard Gwertzman, Russians seem to smoke more and worry about it less, *The New York Times*, Dec. 27, 1970, p. 47.
119. Rosenberg (Ed.), op. cit., p. 44.
120. Psychotherapeutic drug use in USA reported by NIMH scientists, *HEW News*, mimeographed, Apr. 4, 1972, p. 2.
121. France calls addicts diseased, *Hospital Tribune*, Sept. 21, 1970, p. 1.
122. United Nations, op. cit., pp. 125, 225, 226, 228.
123. The new Public Enemy No. 1, *Time*, June 28, 1971, p. 18.
124. News and comment: City-sponsored health research eludes New York budget axe, *Science*, 173:1108 (Sept. 17), 1971.
125. No check in world smoking epidemic, *Sunday Telegraph* (London), Jan. 10, 1971, p. 1.
126. Patricia M. Wald et al. (Eds.), *Dealing with Drug Abuse*, p. 257.
127. Quoted in Rosenberg (Ed.), op. cit., pp. 319, 325.
128. Quoted in *U. S. News and World Report*, April 3, 1972, p. 38.
129. Restrictions proposed on barbiturate sales, *Syracuse Herald-Journal*, Nov. 17, 1972, p. 2.
130. $1 billion voted for drug fight, *Syracuse Herald-Journal*, March 16, 1972, p. 32.
131. Ronald Smothers, Muslims: What's behind the violence, *The New York Times*, Dec. 26, 1972, p. 38.
132. Italian law would treat addiction as a sickness, *The New York Times*, Dec. 24, 1972, p. 18.
133. Wald et al. (Eds.), op. cit., p. 28.
134. Frances Lewine, Nixon focuses on drug fight, *Syracuse Herald-Journal*, March 20, 1972, p. 1.
135. The nation, *American Medical News*, May 21, 1973, p. 2.
136. George Gallup, Life for pushers, *Syracuse Herald-American*, Feb. 11, 1973, p. 78.
137. Quoted in Andrew H. Malcolm, Drug raids terrorize 2 families—by mistake, *The New York Times*, April 29, 1973, pp. 1, 43; p. 43.
138. Rocky signs anti-drug bill, *Syracuse Post-Standard*, May 9, 1973, p. 3.
139. Michael R. Sonnenreich, Discussion of the Final Report of the National Commission on Marijuana and Drug Abuse, *Villanova Law Review*, 18:817–827 (May), 1973; p. 818.

ADDENDUM TO THE APPENDIX

140. Albaugh, B.J. and Anderson, P.O., "Peyote in the treatment of alcoholism among American Indians," *American Journal of Psychiatry*, 131: 1247-1250 (November), 1974; p. 1247.
141. Brody, J.E., "Heavy smoking called disorder," *The New York Times*, June 5, 1975, p. 38.
142. "3 Carter sons told mother of drug use," *The New York Times*, September 3, 1976, p. A-12.
143. Murphy-Ferris, J.T.M. and Torrey, L., "The apricot connection," *New Scientist* (London), June 30, 1977, pp. 766-768; p. 766.
144. "Forms on U.S. contracts reminded to hire alcoholics, drug abusers," *International Herald-Tribune*, July 7, 1977, p. 4.
145. Szasz, T.S., *The Therapeutic State* (Buffalo, N.Y.: Prometheus Books, 1974), pp. 284-296.
146. "People," *International Herald-Tribune*, September 7, 1979, p. 16.
147. "People," *International Herald-Tribune*, January 21, 1980, p. 16.
148. Greenspan, A., "Gold-chain grabbers? Carey blames Soviet heroin-war strategy," *New York Post*, September 26, 1980, p. 10.
149. Seaberry, J., "Japan lifts import duties on tobacco," *Washington Post*, November 22, 1980, p. C-1.
150. "People," *International Herald-Tribune*, December 17, 1980, p. 16.
151. Herman, R., "Carey would sip a glass of PCBs," *The New York Times*, March 5, 1981, p. B-2.
152. See Szasz, T.S., "The protocols of the learned experts on heroin," *Libertarian Review*, July, 1981, pp. 297-303.
153. "Risky rendezvous at Swatow," *Time*, October 19, 1981, p. 109.
154. Howe, M., "Turkey, with kerchief ban, raises Islamic outcry," *The New York Times*, December 19, 1981, p. A-4.
155. "Supreme Court roundup: 40-year term held 'legislative prerogative,' " *The New York Times*, January 13, 1982, p. B-15.
156. Hume, E., "Sniffing paint gets man 2-year jail term," *Ithaca Journal*, February 11, 1982, p. 29.
157. "Just ask your children," *New York Post*, March 10, 1982, p. 24.
158. "Goldwater says his son smoked pot, sniffed coke," *Pittsburgh Press*, April 22, 1983, p. A-27.
159. Werner, L.M., "Agency sells drug kit, then arrests buyer," *The New York Times*, August 11, 1983, p. A-1.
160. "NYC ex-mayor's son is jailed," *Syracuse Herald-Journal*, October 1, 1983, p. A-9.
161. Brown, N., "Doctor willing to defy condom law again," *The Irish Times*, December 9, 1983, p. 2.
162. "Unkosher crop big Israeli export item," *Syracuse Post-Standard*, December 29, 1983, p. C-5.
163. "Robert Kennedy, Jr. admits he is guilty on heroin count," *The New York Times*, February 18, 1964, p. A-8.
164. "Koch urges death penalty for drug dealers," *Syracuse Herald-Journal*, May 1, 1984, p. A-2.
165. "New drug rule takes effect at Massachusetts school," *The Washington Post*, Sept. 8, 1984, p. A-16.

Bibliography

References to articles, reports, and other items appearing in journals, magazines, newspapers, and pamphlets are fully identified in the References; books cited in the References only by author and title are identified more completely below.

Basler, R. P. (Ed.). *The Collected Works of Abraham Lincoln.* New Brunswick, N.J.: Rutgers University Press, 1953.

Bates, M. *Gluttons and Libertines: Human Problems of Being Natural* [1958]. New York: Vintage, 1971.

Breastead, M. *Oh! Sex Education!* New York: Signet, 1971.

Brecher, E. M., et al. *Licit and Illicit Drugs: The Consumers Union Report on Narcotics, Stimulants, Depressants, Inhalants, Hallucinogens, and Marijuana—Including Caffeine, Nicotine, and Alcohol.* Boston: Little, Brown, 1972.

Burke, E. *The Works of the Right Honorable Edmund Burke.* Boston: Wells & Lilly, 1826.

Canadian Government's Commission of Inquiry. *The Non-Medical Uses of Drugs: Interim Report.* Harmondsworth, Eng.: Penguin, 1971.

Catlin, G. E. G. *Liquor Control.* London: Thornton Butterworth, 1931.

Chesler, P. *Women and Madness.* Garden City, N.Y.: Doubleday, 1972.

Crafts, Dr. and Mrs. W. F., and Leitch, M. and M. W. *Intoxicating Drinks and Drugs, in All Lands and Times: A Twentieth Century Survey of Intemperance, Based on a Symposium of Testimony from One Hundred Missionaries and Travelers.* Washington, D.C.: International Reform Bureau, 1900.

Dahmus, J. H. *The Prosecution of John Wyclyf.* New Haven: Yale University Press, 1952.

De Quincey, T. *Confessions of an English Opium Eater* [1822]. Edited with an Introduction by Alethea Hayter. Harmondsworth, Eng.: Penguin, 1971.

Douglas, M. *Purity and Danger: An Analysis of Concepts of Pollution and Taboo.* Harmondsworth, Eng.: Pelican, 1970.

Flexner, E. *Century of Struggle: The Woman's Rights Movement in the United States.* New York: Atheneum, 1972.

Forbes, T. R. *The Midwife and the Witch.* New Haven: Yale University Press, 1966.

Fort, J. *The Pleasure Seekers: The Drug Crisis, Youth, and Society.* Indianapolis and New York: Bobbs-Merrill, 1969.

Frazer, J. G. *The Golden Bough: A Study in Magic and Religion* [1922]. One-Volume, Abridged Edition. New York: Macmillan, 1942.

Furst, P. T. (Ed.). *Flesh of the Gods: The Ritual Use of Hallucinogens.* New York: Praeger, 1972.

Gillouin, R. *Man's Hangman Is Man.* Trans. by Dorothy D. Lachman. Mundelein, Ill.: Island Press, 1957.

Goode, E. *Drugs in American Society.* New York: Knopf, 1972.

Goodman, L. S., and Gilman, A. (Eds.). *The Pharmacological Basis of Therapeutics: A Textbook of Pharmacology, Toxicology, and Therapeutics for Physicians and Medical Students.* Fourth Edition. New York: Macmillan, 1970.

Guttmacher, M. S. *Sex Offenses.* New York: Norton, 1951.

Haggard, H. W. *Devils, Drugs, and Doctors: The Story of the Science of Healing from Medicine-Man to Doctor* [1929]. New York: Pocket Books, 1959.

Harrison, J. E. *Epilegomena to the Study of Greek Religion and Themis: A Study of the Social Origins of Greek Religion* [1912, 1921]. New Hyde Park, N.Y.: University Books, 1962.

Hays, H. R. *The Dangerous Sex: The Myth of Feminine Evil.* New York: Putnam, 1964.

Heer, F. *The Intellectual History of Europe* [1953]. Trans. by Jonathan Steinberg. Garden City, N.Y.: Doubleday Anchor, 1968.

Hesse, E. *Narcotics and Drug Addiction.* Trans. by Frank Gaynor. New York: Philosophical Library, 1946.

Hoffer, A., and Osmond, H. *New Hope for Alcoholics.* New Hyde Park, N.Y.: University Books, 1968.

Hole, C. *Witchcraft in England* [1947]. New York: Collier, 1966.

Hunter, W. C. *Bits of Old China.* London: Kegan Paul, Trench & Co., 1885.

Jones, E. *The Life and Work of Sigmund Freud,* Vol. 1. New York: Basic Books, 1953.

Kaplan, J. *Marijuana: The New Prohibition* [1970]. New York: Pocket Books, 1972.

Kessel, N., and Walton, H. *Alcoholism.* Baltimore: Penguin, 1965.

King, R. *The Drug Hang-up: America's Fifty-Year Folly.* New York: Viking, 1972.

Kolb, L. *Drug Addiction: A Medical Problem.* Springfield, Ill.: Charles C Thomas, 1962.

Laurie, P. *Drugs: Medical, Psychological, and Social Facts.* Baltimore: Penguin, 1969.

Lawson, J. C. *Modern Greek Folklore and Ancient Greek Religion: A Study of Survivals.* Cambridge, Eng.: Cambridge University Press, 1910.

Lindesmith, A. R. *The Addict and the Law.* Bloomington, Ind.: Indiana University Press, 1965.

——. *Addiction and Opiates.* Chicago: Aldine, 1968.

Long, L. H. (Ed.). *The World Almanac and Book of Facts.* 1972 ed. New York: Newspaper Enterprise Association, 1972.

Lyons, J. *Experience: An Introduction to a Personal Psychology.* New York: Harper & Row, 1973.

Mackay, C. *Extraordinary Popular Delusions and the Madness of Crowds* [1841, 1852]. New York: Noonday, 1962.

Malcolm X. *The Autobiography of Malcolm X.* New York: Grove Press, 1966.

Marwick, M. (Ed.). *Witchcraft and Sorcery: Selected Readings.* Harmondsworth, Eng.: Penguin, 1970.

Maudsley, H. *Responsibility in Mental Disease.* Fourth Edition. London: Kegan Paul, Trench & Co., 1885.

Mencken, H. L. *Prejudices: A Selection* (Made by James T. Farrell.) New York: Vintage, 1958.

Menninger, K. *The Vital Balance: The Life Process in Mental Health and Illness.* New York: Viking, 1963.

Michelet, J. *Satanism and Witchcraft: A Study in Medieval Superstition* [1862]. Trans. by A. R. Allinson. New York: Citadel, 1965.

Middleton, J. (Ed.). *Magic, Witchcraft, and Curing.* Garden City, N.Y.: Natural History Press, 1967.

Mises, L. von. *Human Action: A Treatise on Economics.* New Haven: Yale University Press, 1949.

Murray, G. *The Rise of the Greek Epic.* Third Edition. Oxford: Clarendon Press, 1924.

Murray, M. A. *The Witch-Cult in Western Europe* [1921]. Oxford: Oxford Paperbacks, 1962.

Musto, D. F. *The American Disease: Origins of Narcotic Control.* New Haven: Yale University Press, 1973.

Nilsson, M. P. *A History of Greek Religion.* Trans. by F. J. Fielden. Oxford: Clarendon Press, 1925.

Physicians' Desk Reference. 27th Edition. Oradell, N.J.: Medical Economics, 1973.

Rosenberg, S. S. (Ed.). *Alcohol and Health: Report from the Secretary of Health, Education, and Welfare.* New York: Scribner's, 1972.

Roueché, B. *The Neutral Spirit: A Portrait of Alcohol.* Boston: Little, Brown, 1960.

Ryle, G. *The Concept of Mind.* London: Hutchinson's University Library, 1949.

Sartre, J.-P. *Saint Genet: Actor and Martyr* (1952). Trans. by Bernard Frechtman. New York: Braziller, 1963.

Sinclair, A. *Era of Excess: A Social History of the Prohibition Movement.* New York: Harper-Colophon, 1964.

Snyder, S. H. *Uses of Marijuana.* New York: Oxford University Press, 1971.

Solomon, D. (Ed.). *The Marihuana Papers.* New York: Signet, 1968.

Statistical Abstracts of the United States, 1971. 92nd Annual Edition. Washington, D.C.: U. S. Government Printing Office, 1972.

Stevenson, B. (Ed.). *The Macmillan Book of Proverbs, Maxims, and Famous Phrases.* New York: Macmillan, 1948.

Storrs, R. S. *John Wycliffe and the English Bible: An Oration.* New York: Anson D. F. Randolph Co., 1880.

Strauss, M. B. (Ed.). *Familiar Medical Quotations.* Boston: Little, Brown, 1968.

Szasz, T. S. *The Myth of Mental Illness: Foundations of a Theory of Personal Conduct.* New York: Hoeber-Harper, 1961.

——. *Law, Liberty, and Psychiatry: An Inquiry into the Social Uses of Mental Health Practices.* New York: Macmillan, 1963.

——. *Psychiatric Justice.* New York: Macmillan, 1965.

——. *The Ethics of Psychoanalysis: The Theory and Method of Autonomous Psychotherapy.* New York: Basic Books, 1965.

——. *Ideology and Insanity: Essays on the Psychiatric Dehumanization of Man.* Garden City, N.Y.: Doubleday Anchor, 1970.

——. *The Manufacture of Madness: A Comparative Study of the Inquisition and the Mental Health Movement.* New York: Harper & Row, 1970.

——. *The Second Sin.* Garden City, N.Y.: Doubleday, 1973.

——. (Ed.). *The Age of Madness: A History of Involuntary Mental Hospitalization Presented in Selected Texts.* Garden City, N.Y.: Doubleday Anchor, 1973.

Thomas, K. *Religion and the Decline of Magic: Studies in Popular Beliefs in Sixteenth and Seventeenth Century England.* London: Weidenfeld and Nicholson, 1971.

United Nations. *Statistical Yearbook, 1970.* New York: United Nations Publishing Service, 1971.

——. *Statistical Yearbook, 1971.* New York: United Nations Publishing Service, 1972.

Wald, P. M., Hutt, P. B., and DeLong, J. V. (Eds.). *Dealing with Drug Abuse: A Report to the Ford Foundation.* New York: Praeger, 1972. (Copyright 1972, Ford Foundation.)

Wilson, E. *The American Earthquake: A Documentary of the Twenties and Thirties.* Garden City, N.Y.: Doubleday Anchor, 1958.

Wilson, N. L. (Ed.). *Obesity.* Philadelphia: F. A. Davis, 1969.

World Health Organization. *Treatment of Drug Addicts: A Survey of Existing Legislation.* Geneva: World Health Organization, 1962.

Young, J. *The Drugtakers: The Social Meaning of Drug Use.* London: Paladin, 1972.

Zilboorg, G. *A History of Medical Psychology.* New York: Norton, 1941.

INDEX

Nargeolet, Henri, 209
National Academy of Sciences, 140
National Institute of Mental Health, 66–67
Nazis (Nazism), 16, 20, 70, 76–77, 79, 80, 125, 131
Negroes, xviii, 7, 10, 75, 89–103, 112, 195–96; drug use and racism and, 89–103, 112; use of term, 7
"New Drug Offers Hope: May Immunize Heroin Addicts" (Stout), 13, 213
New Testament, 42, 184, 185. See also Bible, the
New York Academy of Medicine, 129, 150
New York State, war against drug use in, 14–16, 20, 21–22, 68, 70, 71–74, 132, 205, 212; drug law (1973), 14–16, 20, 21–22; Narcotics Addiction Control Program (1967), 205
New York Times, The, 13, 15, 46–47, 55, 71–73, 132–33, 204–5
Nicotine, 55, 144, 202. See also Smoking; Tobacco; specific forms
Nidetch, Mrs. Jean, 204
Nietzsche, 29–30
Nilsson, Martin, 24–25
Nixon (Richard M.) administration, 56, 79, 129, 132, 133, 208, 209, 211
Noah (Bible), 41–42
Numbers, Book of, 42

Obedience, authority versus autonomy and, 175–81
Obesity, 93, 105–21; as foodaholism, 105–21; self-control versus social control and, 163–64, 169, 174; surgical treatment for, 116–21
"Obesity: A Gross National Product" (University of California Medical Center symposium, 1967), 109
Ointments, use in religions of, 63–64
Old Testament, 42, 184. See also Bible, the

Oman, J. Campbell, 43
Opiates, 6, 49, 75–87, 130–31 ff., 137–51, 158. See also specific kinds
Opium, 17, 20, 23, 30, 32, 34, 45, 46–51, 55–56, 65, 75–81, 86, 210; chronological history of use and prohibition of, 183–92 passim, 194, 195–96, 202, 203, 210; as a panacea, 130, 131, 138, 140, 141, 142, 143, 145, 150; persecution of Chinese-Americans for use of, 75–81
Opium Conventions, 196; first international, 196
Orientals, American, persecution of opium users among, 75–81
Original sin, 138, 173. See also Adam and Eve; Serpent, the
Orwell, George, 154
Osler, Sir William, 84
Osmond, Humphry, 206

Pain-killing drugs, 3, 65. See also specific kinds
Panaceas, panapathogens and, 26–27, 78, 85, 137–51, 180–81; principal (listed), 138
Pan-American Coffee Bureau, 200–1
Panapathogens. See Panaceas, panapathogens and
Paracelsus, 63, 185
Parade (magazine), 114
Parafon Forte, 150
Parsons, Benjamin, 189
Paton, W. R., 26, 214
Payne, J. Howard, 117–18
Penicillin, 144, 145
Personal Liberty League, 191–92
Petey, George E., 194–95
Peyote, use of, 126–29, 198–99
Phalen, Colonel J. M., 201
Pharmacological Basis of Therapeutics, The, 9, 130–31
Pharmacology, xviii–xix, 3, 8–10, 19, 20, 26, 27, 32; difference between pharmacracy and, 140, 143, 147–48; medicine as magic and, 61–

74; medicine as social control and, 125–36, 137–51 ff.
Pharmacracy, 138, 139–51
Pharmakos (*pharmakoi*), 19–20, 24–27
Phenobarbital, 196
Physicians, xix–xx (*see also* Medicine; Psychiatry; specific aspects, individuals, organizations); and discovery of drug problem, 3–18; drugs as scapegoat and, 21–27 (*see also* Scapegoats); and licit and illicit healing (medicine as magic), 61–74; and medicine as religion, 29–37; and medicine as social control, 125–26, 137–51, 153–74, 175–81; and war against drugs, 21–27, 29–37, 61–74, 87, 125–36, 137–51, 153–74; and war on obesity, 108–21
Physician's Desk Reference (1973), 109
Pills, birth-control, 207
Pipe smoking, 45
"Plague," drug addiction as, xvii, 13, 17, 19, 35, 51, 128
Pleasures, temptation and self-control and, 157–74, 175–81
Plutarch, 23
Pocahontas, 186
Poison(ing), 19, 69
Politics (politicians), and addiction, xiii, 6, 14–17, 54, 74, 103; and drugs as scapegoat, 19–27; and medicine as religion, 30–31, 33; and medicine as social control, 125–36, 137–51, 153–54, 155, 175–81
Pollution and purification, 26–27, 89 ff. *See also* Purification and pollution theme
Poppy, 46–50, 55–56, 65, 183, 201, 210. *See also* Opium
Pork eating, 23, 32–33, 35, 91–92, 94, 98, 185
Possession, demonic, 172
Power (*see also* Authority): anti-drug war and, 86–87, 93; tempta-

tion and social control versus self-control and, 157–58, 169, 175–81
Prayer, 62
Prentice, Alfred C., 99–100, 199
Priest-physicians, 62, 65–66, 67
"Primitive man," drugs as scapegoat and, 19–27
Prohibition(s): alcohol, 32, 36, 113, 127, 135, 184, 185, 186–90, 191–94 *passim*, 208; chronological history of addiction and, 183–212; defiance of authority and, 169–74, 175–81; drugs as scapegoat and, 22–27, 29; of drugs, 22–27, 29 ff., 46–57, 61–64, 75–87, 125–36, 137–51, 169–74, 183–212 *passim* (*see also* Drug laws; specific drugs, laws); medicine as magic and, 61–74; medicine as religion and, 29–37; medicine as social control and, 125–36, 137–51
Prohibition Party, 191
Projections, psychological, 77
Proverbs (Bible), 184
Psalms, Book of, 184
Psychiatry (psychiatrists), xviii; and addiction, xviii, 3, 4–8, 9–12, 16–18, 33–34, 53–54, 69, 125–36, 137–51, 153–74, 176–81; and drug control as social control, 125–36, 137–51, 153–74, 176–81; and drugs as scapegoat, 21–27, 53–54, 76; and medicine and science as religion, 33–34; and obesity, 107, 110, 116, 119
Psychoactive drugs, 14, 32, 63–64 ff., 82, 148, 209. *See also* Mood-affecting drugs; specific kinds
Psychology, 5, 166, 177–78 (*see also* Psychiatry); and social control, 153–54
Puerto Ricans, xviii
Pure Food and Drug Act, first, 195
Purification and pollution theme, 26–27, 89 ff.; drug control and, 125, 137–51; drugs as scapegoat and, 26–27, 89 ff.; panaceas and panapathogens and, 137–51;

weight control and, 105, 106–7, 111–12, 119
Puritans, Black Muslims and, 94
"Pushers," xiii–xv, xviii, 6, 14–16, 64, 66, 70–74, 79; drugs as scapegoat and, 20, 26, 79, 142, 147, 159, 165, 167–69, 176, 179, 180

Racism, addiction and, 75–81, 83–103
Ramirez, Dr. Efren, 206
Religion (see also specific aspects, religions): ceremonial drug use as communion and, 39–57; Communism and, 146–47; drugs as scapegoat and, 19–27, 29; medicine as, 61–74, 105–21 passim, 125–36 passim, 153, 154, 156, 158, 160, 161, 162, 171–72; medicine as science and, 3–18, 21, 29–37, 96; and medicine as social control, 125–36, 137–51 passim, 154, 156, 160, 161, 162–72; and panaceas, 137–51; and war against drugs, xiii, xiv, xviii, xix–xx, 3–5, 11, 17, 19–27, 29, 61–74, 85–87, 89–103
Rensenberger, Boyce, 13, 213
Responsibility, social control and, 138, 159, 160, 170–74, 176, 178
Retreat for the Insane (Hartford, Conn.), 7
Ritual(ism): ceremonial drug use and, 39–57; drugs as scapegoat and, 19–27, 29; medicine as religion and, 29–37
Robespierre, 177
Rockefeller, Nelson A., 14–16, 71–74, 79, 132, 205, 212
Rolfe, John, 186
Rolleston, J. D., 184–85
Rush, Benjamin, 95, 96, 177, 187–88
Russia. See Soviet Union (Russia)

"Sabbat," celebration of, 63
Saccharin, 140, 143
"Saccharin Suspect in Study," 140
Sacrifice: drugs as scapegoat and, 19–27, 29, 35–36; temptation and

self-control versus social control and, 156–74
Saint Genet (Sartre), 90
Saleh, Dr. Jehanshaw, 50–51
Sanders, Marion, 56, 216
Sandman, C. W., Jr., 205
Santayana, George, 96
Sartre, Jean-Paul, 90
Scapegoats (scapegoating), addiction and, 19–27, 55; drug use and, xiii–xiv, xv, 19–27, 29, 55, 61–74, 75–83, 92, 137, 142; obesity and, 105–21
Schizophrenia, xvii, 7, 117, 172
Schless, Robert A., 199
Schoeck, Helmut, 168
Science (magazine), 12
Science, and addiction, xiv–xv, xviii, xx, 3–18, 19–27, 61–74, 87, 96, 140; drugs as scapegoat and, 19–27, 87; magic and medicine as religion and, 3–18, 30–37, 61–74, 96, 105 (see also Magic; Medicine; Religion); and medicine as social control, 125–36, 137–51, 153–74, 175, 181; scientism and, xiv–xv, 140
Self-control, addiction and social control versus, 35, 44, 137–51, 154–74, 175–81
Self-determination, authority versus, 175–81
Sennett, William C., 133
Serpent, the, 86, 167. See also Adam and Eve
Sertürner, Friedrich Wilhelm Adam, 189
Sex (sexual activity), 95, 106–7, 129–30, 142, 180, 197 (see also Homosexuality; Masturbation); alcohol use and, 197; social control versus self-control and temptation and, 157–58, 160–62, 168, 169, 170, 180
Shabazz (tribe), 97, 101
Shabazz, El Hajj Melik, 101
Shafer, Raymond P., 132–34
Shakespeare, William, 185
Sixteenth Amendment, 196